Department of Veterans Affairs
Health Services Research & Development Service | Evidence-based Synthesis Program

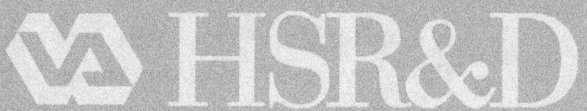

I0470860

# Management of Inpatient Hyperglycemia: A Systematic Review

October 2008

## Prepared for:

Department of Veterans Affairs
Veterans Health Administration
Health Services Research & Development Service
Washington, DC 20420

## Investigators:

Devan Kansagara, MD
*Principal Investigator*

Fawn Wolf, MD
*Investigator*

Michele Freeman, MPH
*Research Associate*

Mark Helfand, MD, MPH
*Director*

## Prepared by:

Portland Veterans Affairs Healthcare System
Oregon Evidence-based Practice Center
Portland, OR

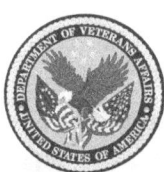

# PREFACE

VA's Health Services Research and Development Service (HSR&D) works to improve the cost, quality, and outcomes of health care for our nation's veterans. Collaborating with VA leaders, managers, and policy makers, HSR&D focuses on important health care topics that are likely to have significant impact on quality improvement efforts. One significant collaborative effort is HSR&D's Evidence-based Synthesis Program (ESP). Through this program, HSR&D provides timely and accurate evidence syntheses on targeted health care topics. These products will be disseminated broadly throughout VA and will: inform VA clinical policy, develop clinical practice guidelines, set directions for future research to address gaps in knowledge, identify the evidence to support VA performance measures, and rationalize drug formulary decisions.

HSR&D provided funding for the two Evidence Based Practice Centers (EPCs) supported by the Agency for Healthcare Research and Quality (AHRQ) that also had an active and publicly acknowledged VA affiliation – Southern California EPC and Portland, OR EPC – so they could develop evidence syntheses on requested topics for dissemination to VA policymakers. A planning committee with representation from HSR&D, Patient Care Services, Office of Quality and Performance, and the VISN Clinical Management Officers, has been established to identify priority topics and to insure the quality of final reports.

Comments on this evidence report are welcome and can be sent to Susan Schiffner, ESP Program Manager, at Susan.Schiffner@va.gov.

# EXECUTIVE SUMMARY

## BACKGROUND

Hyperglycemia is a common finding in hospitalized patients and has been associated with worsened outcomes in a variety of inpatient subpopulations. The use of insulin to control blood glucose has been advocated as a way to improve health outcomes in hospitalized patients with hyperglycemia, but the evidence for the efficacy of this approach and the thresholds for initiating insulin management are unclear.

The key questions were:

1. Does strict blood glucose control compared to less strict blood glucose control improve final health outcomes in the following patients?
   - patients in the medical intensive care unit
   - patients in the surgical intensive care unit
   - acute myocardial infarction patients
   - acute stroke patients
   - post coronary artery bypass graft patients
   - general surgical ward patients
   - general medicine ward patients

2. What are the harms of strict blood glucose control in the above subpopulations?

3. What are the most effective and safest means of normalizing blood glucose in the above subpopulations?

## METHODS

We conducted searches in Medline and the Cochrane database of systematic reviews of literature published from 1950 through May 2008, and obtained additional articles from systematic reviews, reference lists of pertinent studies, reviews, editorials, and by consulting experts. We also searched for information about unpublished studies on clinicaltrials.gov and included these studies if the authors provided enough detail to enable quality rating. Reviewers trained in the critical analysis of literature assessed for relevance the abstracts of citations identified from literatures searches. Full-text articles of potentially relevant abstracts were retrieved for further review. We assessed the overall quality of evidence for outcomes by considering the consistency, coherence, and applicability of a body of evidence, as well as the internal validity of individual studies, using a method developed by the Grade Working Group.(1) We performed a meta-analysis of trials conducted in critical care settings to estimate the effects of achieving normoglycemia using intensive insulin therapy on short-term mortality and risk of hypoglycemia.

# RESULTS

We reviewed 2313 titles and abstracts from the electronic search, an additional 44 from reference mining and recently published studies, and also 9 unpublished studies. We retrieved 356 full-text articles for further review. We included 26 RCTs and 3 systematic reviews in synthesizing evidence for key question 1. For key question 2, we evaluated the results of 23 RCTs, 2 systematic reviews, and 10 studies that were either observational studies or trials without health outcomes. To address key question 3, we included 3 systematic reviews and 2 RCTs, as well as the 10 observational studies and trials without health outcomes.

## KEY QUESTION #1. Does strict glycemic control compared to less strict glycemic control improve final health outcomes in the following patients?

Very little intervention data is available to help clearly define a glucose threshold that should prompt glucose lowering efforts in various inpatient subpopulations. The benefits of achieving normoglycemia with aggressive insulin use are inconsistent and may be limited to subgroups of critically ill patients receiving aggressive nutrition and in whom reliable glucose monitoring methods are used. Use of insulin to achieve normoglycemia is associated with a considerable risk of hypoglycemia. Higher glucose targets can likely be relatively safely achieved in inpatients, though the impact of this practice on health outcomes is uncertain.

### Patients in Medical and Surgical Intensive Care Units

We found eight unblinded randomized, controlled trials examining the efficacy of tight glycemic control using intensive insulin regimens in critically ill patients, including two in the medical ICU (MICU) setting, two in the surgical ICU (SICU) setting, and four in mixed MICU/SICU settings. Single-center evidence had initially shown a mortality and morbidity benefit from IIT in subgroups of patients requiring prolonged ICU stays, but the applicability of these data to other ICUs may be limited and subsequent trials have not confirmed this benefit. Our meta-analysis found the use of intensive insulin therapy to achieve normoglycemia had a neutral effect on short-term mortality, but increased the risk of hypoglycemia more than five-fold. (GRADE: Moderate = further research is likely to have an important impact on our confidence in the estimate of effect and may change the estimate.)

### Acute Myocardial Infarction Patients

We found good evidence that insulin used as part of a fixed-dose glucose-insulin-potassium infusion does not consistently improve final health outcomes in acute myocardial infarction patients, and may increase short-term mortality. (GRADE: High = Further research is unlikely to change our confidence on the estimate of effect.)

Six trials have examined tight glycemic control using adjustable dose insulin-based regimens. As a body of evidence, these studies fail to demonstrate consistent evidence of the benefits of adjustable dose insulin-based regimens in acute myocardial infarction patients, but variation in trial design, achievement of recruitment goals, glucose level achieved, and concomitant therapy for myocardial infarction limit the strength of this conclusion. (GRADE: Low = Further research is very likely to have an important impact on our confidence in the estimate of effect and may change the estimate.)

## Acute Stroke Patients

The largest trial to date in stroke patients reported largely negative results, but was hampered by low participation rates and incomplete data reporting. A second much smaller fair-quality trial in patients with subarachnoid hemorrhage failed to find a long-term clinical benefit from tight glycemic control, but did find a reduced infection rate in the short-term. Thus there is very little good-quality evidence investigating tight glycemic control in patients who have suffered a cerebrovascular accident. (GRADE: Low = Further research is very likely to have an important impact on our confidence in the estimate of effect and may change the estimate.)

## Post Coronary Artery Bypass Graft Patients and General Surgical Ward Patients

We found five trials which varied widely in design, blood glucose levels attained, and in the inclusion of patients with diabetes, limiting the comparability of results across studies. Several studies were underpowered to evaluate the outcomes of interest in this review. Neither insulin infusion nor GIK infusion given perioperatively provided a clear benefit among cardiac surgery patients in any of the studies. One good-quality meta-analysis reviewed a diverse group of GIK and insulin infusion studies in peri- and postoperative settings and found largely negative results when the largest trial (reviewed under the ICU section above) was excluded.

Overall, there is no clear evidence showing a benefit of tight glycemic control strategies in the perioperative setting, but the trial evidence is methodologically limited. (GRADE: low = Further research is likely to have an important impact on our confidence in the estimate of effect and is likely to change the estimate.)

## General Medicine Ward Patients

There were no studies evaluating a tight glycemic control strategy to less tight glycemic control in general medical ward patients. Thus, the overall level of evidence in this subpopulation is very low (GRADE: Very Low = Any estimate of effect is very uncertain.)

## KEY QUESTION #2. What are the harms of strict blood glucose control in the above subpopulations?

There is a considerable risk of hypoglycemia in medical ICU patients treated with intensive insulin protocols designed to normalize blood glucose. This risk was lower in surgical ICU patients receiving similar therapy, and in myocardial infarction, stroke, and perioperative patients in whom the target glucose level was generally not aimed at strict normoglycemia. Data from numerous mainly single-center observational studies and trials not examining health outcomes suggest the incidence of hypoglycemia may be considerably lower when less strict glucose targets are used. There was very little evidence that hypoglycemia from tight glycemic control protocols resulted in short-term adverse health outcomes, but the long-term effects of inpatient hypoglycemia have not been well studied.

## KEY QUESTION #3. What are the most effective and safest means of normalizing blood glucose in the above subpopulations?

A number of insulin infusion protocols (IIPs) have been evaluated, but comparative effectiveness data are lacking. The protocols differed in terms of patient characteristics, target glucose ranges, the time required to achieve the target glucose, the incidence and definition of hypoglycemia, the rationale or algorithm used for adjusting the insulin rates, the methods used to assess effectiveness and the methods of glucose monitoring. Given this variety of factors, reviewers have suggested each institution should individualize its approach to protocol implementation based on its patient population as well as its institutional and provider resources. Based on comparisons across studies, some reviewers speculate better protocols incorporate bolus insulin doses, account for the direction and rate of glucose change, and make allowances for "off-protocol" adjustments, although this conclusion is not based on direct comparisons of protocols.

Basal bolus subcutaneous insulin regimens may be more effective in lowering blood glucose than sliding scale regimens, though there is very limited evidence comparing methods of blood glucose control in ward patients.

# TABLE OF CONTENTS

# BACKGROUND

Hyperglycemia is a common finding among medical and surgical inpatients with and without known diabetes,(2, 3) and is associated with poor outcomes across a variety of inpatient subpopulations.(2, 4-8) The relationship between hyperglycemia and inpatient outcomes may be weaker in patients with diabetes than in patients without diabetes.(9, 10)

Hyperglycemia may be a marker of severe, acute illness, one of many physiological derangements associated with an abundance of counter-regulatory hormones, insulin resistance, and suppression of anabolic pathways.(11) On the other hand, many investigators believe that hyperglycemia itself may worsen outcomes by contributing to inflammation, oxidative stress, poor immune function, and endothelial dysfunction.(12)

Interventions to control hyperglycemia in inpatients have largely centered on the use of adjustable insulin infusions to lower blood glucose. An early trial in myocardial infarction patients found that lowering blood glucose using intensive insulin therapy (IIT) reduced long-term mortality, though it remains unclear whether the inpatient or outpatient components of the intervention were responsible for the benefit.(13) An influential single-center observational study of cardiac surgery patients reported reduced wound infection and mortality rates after the introduction of an intensive care unit IIT protocol.(14, 15) Subsequently a single-center trial in critically ill surgical patients suggested a mortality benefit from IIT used to achieve normoglycemia.(16)

These findings have fueled widespread interest in inpatient glycemic control strategies,(17, 18) and organizations have called for strict glycemic control strategies to be implemented in a variety of intensive care unit settings.(12, 19) More recently, new trials have been completed that may help clarify the balance of benefits and harms of widespread IIT implementation in intensive care units. We conducted a systematic review of trials and a critical appraisal of frequently cited observational studies to identify strengths of—and gaps in—the evidence supporting broad use of IIT to achieve glycemic control in inpatients.

# METHODS

## Topic Development

The review was commissioned by the Department of Veterans Affairs' Evidence-based Synthesis Program. We conferred with VA and non-VA experts to select the patients and subgroups, interventions, outcomes, and setting addressed in the review.

The objectives of this review are to address the following questions:

1. Does the use of intensive insulin therapy (IIT) to achieve tight glycemic control compared to less tight glycemic control improve final health outcomes in the following patients?

- patients in the surgical intensive care unit
- patients in the medical intensive care unit
- patients in the perioperative setting
- acute myocardial infarction patients
- acute stroke patients
- general surgical ward patients
- general medicine ward patients

2. What are the harms of strict glycemic control in the above subpopulations?

3. What are the most effective and safest means of lowering blood glucose in the above subpopulations?

Figure 1 illustrates the analytic framework that guided our review and synthesis.

# Figure 1. Analytic Framework

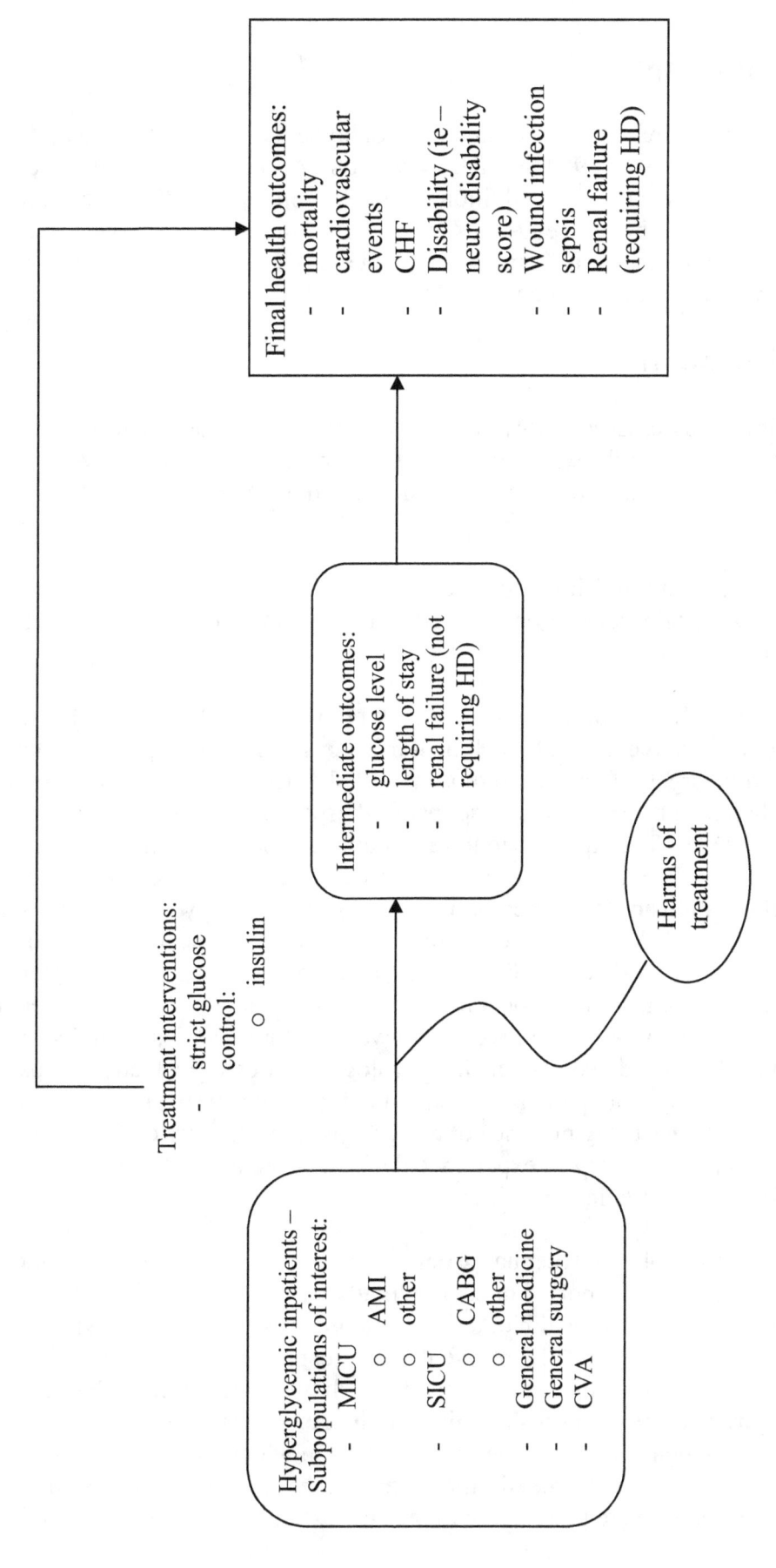

Treatment interventions:
- strict glucose control:
  o insulin

Hyperglycemic inpatients –
Subpopulations of interest:
- MICU
  o AMI
  o other
- SICU
  o CABG
  o other
- General medicine
- General surgery
- CVA

Intermediate outcomes:
- glucose level
- length of stay
- renal failure (not requiring HD)

Harms of treatment

Final health outcomes:
- mortality
- cardiovascular events
- CHF
- Disability (ie – neuro disability score)
- Wound infection
- sepsis
- Renal failure (requiring HD)

3

## Search Strategy

We conducted a search in Medline and the Cochrane database of systematic reviews of literature published from 1950 through May 2008. Appendix A provides the search strategy in detail. We obtained additional articles from systematic reviews, reference lists of pertinent studies, reviews, editorials, and by consulting experts. We also searched for information about unpublished studies on clinicaltrials.gov. All citations were imported into an electronic database (EndNote X1).

## Study Selection

Three reviewers assessed for relevance the abstracts of citations identified from literatures searches. Full-text articles of potentially relevant abstracts were retrieved for further review. Each article retrieved was reviewed using the eligibility criteria shown in Appendix B.

Eligible articles had English-language abstracts and provided primary data relevant to the key questions. Eligibility criteria varied depending on the question of interest, as described below.

To evaluate the efficacy of intensive insulin therapy (IIT) in hospitalized patients, we considered prospective, controlled clinical trials of insulin-based protocols targeted to strict glycemic targets compared to those targeted to less strict glycemic targets. We also considered clinical trials of fixed-dose insulin-based treatment regimens in myocardial infarction patients. The studies had to report at least one prespecified final health outcome (Appendix B). Unpublished studies were included if the authors could provide enough information about the methodology and results to fully evaluate the study's quality. We excluded insulin-based studies conducted in myocardial infarction patients prior to widespread availability of thrombolytics (i.e., enrolling patients prior to 1990).(20) We categorized perioperative trials as those in which IIT was begun pre-, intra-, or immediately post-operatively, and was continued for less than 24 hours post-operatively. We considered patients in neurologic, neurosurgical, and coronary intensive care units separately from patients in general medical and surgical ICUs. Though observational studies using historic control groups were initially excluded from our review, after consultation with experts we decided to include a discussion and critique of frequently cited observational studies.

To assess the risk of hypoglycemia associated with IIT, we included controlled trials and uncontrolled series that reported rates of hypoglycemia in ICU patients treated with IIT, even if they did not report health outcomes. In order to avoid studies with substantial selection bias, we included only interventional prospective cohort studies in which patients were consecutively enrolled and in which there was minimal loss to follow-up. Because tight glycemic control strategies require some personnel training and institutional acceptance, we included only studies in which the intervention was evaluated over a prolonged period of time (defined as 6 months for the purposes of this review) as we felt these studies were most likely to provide externally valid results.

To assess the effectiveness of specific inpatient blood glucose control strategies in lowering blood glucose, we evaluated fair to good quality systematic reviews of insulin infusion protocols. Because of the relative dearth of information guiding insulin management in general medical or surgical ward patients, we also included primary data from controlled clinical trials evaluating subcutaneous insulin management strategies in general medical or surgical ward patients (e.g., those that compared sliding scale insulin to scheduled insulin).

## Data abstraction

From each study we abstracted the following: study design, objectives, setting, population characteristics (including sex, age, baseline morbidity), subject eligibility and exclusion criteria, number of subjects, years of enrollment, duration of follow-up, the study and comparator interventions, the method used to monitor blood glucose, the target range for blood glucose control, the outcomes measured, the analytic method used, the variables adjusted in the analysis, the results of the study and the mean blood glucose achieved in each group, information on concomitant therapy/nutrition, the occurrence of hypoglycemia in each group, and any other adverse events.

## Rating the body of evidence

We assessed the overall quality of evidence for outcomes using a method developed by the Grade Working Group.(1) The Grade method considers the consistency, coherence, and applicability of a body of evidence, as well as the internal validity of individual studies to classify the grade of evidence across outcomes as follows:

High = Further research is very unlikely to change our confidence on the estimate of effect.
Moderate = Further research is likely to have an important impact on our confidence in the estimate of effect and may change the estimate.
Low = Further research is very likely to have an important impact on our confidence in the estimate of effect and is likely to change the estimate.
Very Low = Any estimate of effect is very uncertain.

The quality of each study was rated as good, fair, or poor based on the following criteria: the comparability of treatment groups; the adequacy of randomization; whether treatment allocation was concealed; whether eligibility criteria were specified; the use of blinding among patients, care providers, and outcome assessors; whether the analysis was intention-to-treat, or conducted with post-randomization exclusions, or with extensive or differential loss to follow-up; clearly defined interventions and reliable outcome measurement (Appendix C).(21) When reviewers disagreed, consensus was reached through discussion with all authors.

## Data synthesis

Because all ICU trials except one (22) were either small (n < 100) (23-25) or did not reach recruitment goals (16, 26-29), we performed a meta-analysis of trials conducted in critical care settings to estimate with greater power the effects of achieving normoglycemia using IIT on short-term mortality and hypoglycemia. The clinical heterogeneity of insulin interventions, glucose targets, and population characteristics precluded quantitative analysis within the perioperative, myocardial infarction, and stroke subgroups. We abstracted the number of events and total subjects from each treatment arm, and obtained a pooled estimate of relative risk (RR) using a random effects model.(30) Trials reporting hospital or 28-day mortality were included in the short-term mortality analysis. We performed sensitivity analyses to assess the effects of short-term mortality definition (i.e. hospital or 28 day mortality), as well as the effects of excluding trials using higher intervention glucose targets.

Statistical heterogeneity was assessed by Cochran's Q test and $I^2$ statistic.(31) Because of the small number of trials that could be combined, we did not perform assessments for publication bias.(32) All analyses were performed using Stata 10.0 (StataCorp, College Station, TX, 2007).

## Peer review

A draft version of this report was sent to the technical advisory panel and additional peer reviewers. Their comments and our responses are shown in Appendix D.

# RESULTS

## Literature Flow

We reviewed 2313 titles and abstracts from the electronic search, and identified an additional 44 from reference mining and recently published studies. We also identified 9 unpublished or ongoing studies.(26-28, 33-38) Three of these studies have been completed and the authors provided enough information for us to quality rate and formally include the studies.(26-28)

After applying inclusion/exclusion criteria at the abstract level, 356 full-text articles were reviewed, as shown in Figure 2. Of the full-text articles, we rejected 288 that did not meet our inclusion criteria.

## Figure 2. Management of Inpatient Hyperglycemia Literature Flow

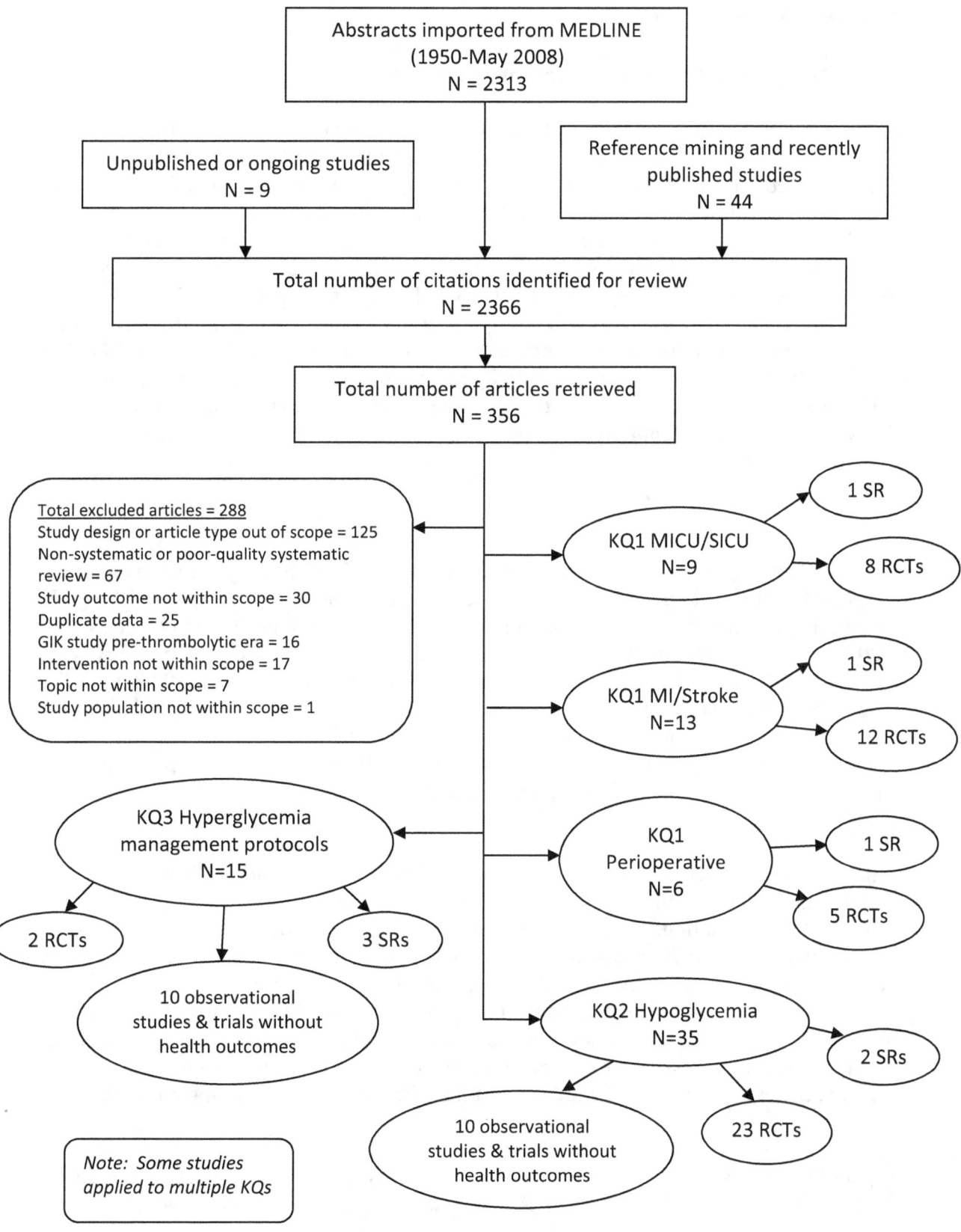

Abstracts imported from MEDLINE
(1950-May 2008)
N = 2313

Unpublished or ongoing studies
N = 9

Reference mining and recently
published studies
N = 44

Total number of citations identified for review
N = 2366

Total number of articles retrieved
N = 356

Total excluded articles = 288
Study design or article type out of scope = 125
Non-systematic or poor-quality systematic
review = 67
Study outcome not within scope = 30
Duplicate data = 25
GIK study pre-thrombolytic era = 16
Intervention not within scope = 17
Topic not within scope = 7
Study population not within scope = 1

KQ1 MICU/SICU
N=9

1 SR

8 RCTs

KQ1 MI/Stroke
N=13

1 SR

12 RCTs

KQ3 Hyperglycemia
management protocols
N=15

KQ1
Perioperative
N=6

1 SR

5 RCTs

2 RCTs

3 SRs

10 observational
studies & trials without
health outcomes

KQ2 Hypoglycemia
N=35

2 SRs

10 observational
studies & trials without
health outcomes

23 RCTs

Note: Some studies
applied to multiple KQs

7

**KEY QUESTION #1.  Does strict glycemic control compared to less strict glycemic control improve final health outcomes in the following patients?**

**Patients in Medical and Surgical Intensive Care Units**

Eight  unblinded randomized, controlled trials evaluated tight glycemic control using intensive insulin therapy (IIT) in critically ill patients (Table 1).(16, 22-24, 26-29)  Two trials included critically ill surgical patients (SICU)(16, 24), two trials included critically ill medical patients (MICU),(22, 23) and four  trials included a mixed SICU/MICU population.(26-29)  All of the trials except for one(23) investigated the relative benefits of glucose targets in the normoglycemic range (80 – 110 mg/dL) compared to moderate glucose targets (140 – 200 mg/dL).  Our combined analysis of all seven ICU studies(16, 22, 24, 26-29) evaluating the use of intensive insulin therapy to achieve normoglycemia found the intervention had a neutral effect on short-term mortality (RR 0.90; 95% CI 0.78 – 1.03, $I^2$ 40.7%; Figure 3), and substantially increased the risk of hypoglycemia (RR 5.32; 95% CI 4.21 – 6.73, $I^2$ 2.28%; Figure 4).(GRADE: Moderate = further research is likely to have an important impact on our confidence in the estimate of effect and may change the estimate).

*SICU*

In one influential trial, Van den Berghe et al randomized 1548 SICU patients to either a simple IIT protocol (Leuven protocol) targeted to normal blood glucose (80 – 110 mg/dL by morning blood glucose), or conventional therapy designed to keep blood glucose 180 – 200 mg/dL.  This study was terminated early after finding all-cause ICU mortality was significantly lower in the intensive insulin group (4.6% v. 8%, relative risk 0.58, 95% CI 0.38-0.78)(Table 1).(16)  The short-term mortality benefit was limited to the subgroup of patients requiring 5 or more days of ICU care (10.6 vs 20.2%, p = 0.005), and long-term mortality did not differ between the two groups.(39)  The intervention group experienced a higher cumulative incidence of hypoglycemia (5% v. 0.76%; RR 6.65, 95 % CI 2.83 – 15.62).

This trial was conducted in a SICU that used intravenous glucose and TPN routinely, and monitored all patients with arterial blood sampling, a more accurate method than capillary blood sampling. These practices are not standard in most SICUs. These characteristics may limit the applicability of these results to nonsurgical patients, patients not receiving parenteral nutrition, and centers mainly relying on capillary blood samples.(40-42)  Given the nature of the intervention and need for frequent monitoring, blinding of care providers was not possible in this or any of the other studies considered. Though outcomes assessors were blinded, it is possible that patients assigned to IIT received better overall management as a result of the intensive monitoring required for IIT.

A poor quality trial conducted among 61 SICU patients found that establishing normal blood glucose levels (80 – 120 mg/dL) compared to a moderate glucose target (180 – 220 mg/dL) in surgical ICU patients using IIT similar to the Leuven protocol was associated with a 4-fold decrease in intravascular device and bloodstream infections (p<0.05), but not a decrease in mortality (Table 1).(24) The study had numerous methodologic flaws including lack of blinding of outcome assessors, poorly defined exclusion criteria, and failure to report numbers of patients excluded and reasons for exclusion.

*MICU*

The mortality benefits seen in Van den Berghe et al's SICU trial have not been replicated in MICU populations.(16) A fair-quality trial by Van den Berghe et al included 1200 adult patients admitted to a single medical ICU.(22) As with the other included trials, blinding of care providers was not feasible and could potentially have resulted in treatment bias. Those who were assumed to require less than three days of intensive care, specifically those who were able to receive oral nutrition, were excluded. The methods, insulin regimens and glucose targets were similar to Van den Berghe's 2001 surgical ICU study, but both arterial and capillary blood samples were used in this study for glucose monitoring. Patients received just over 1200 kcal/day of nutritional support in both groups and the vast majority received most nutrition parenterally. Neither in-hospital nor ICU mortality was reduced in the overall intention to treat population, but in-hospital mortality was reduced from 52.5% to 43% (relative risk 0.82, 95% CI not given, p=0.009) in the prespecified subgroup of patients staying in the ICU for at least a third day. There was a nonsignificant mortality increase associated with intensive therapy (relative risk 1.09, 95% CI 0.9-1.32) amongst the 433 patients requiring less than 3 days of ICU care. The incidence of hypoglycemia was significantly higher in the intervention group (Table 4) and mortality was non-significantly higher among those who experienced at least one episode of hypoglycemia (66.7% v. 46.4%, p = 0.1).

A small, poor quality trial in a single MICU examined the efficacy of targeting more moderate glucose goals: 110-140 mg/dl in the intensive group and 140-200 in the control group.(23) Neither ICU nor one month mortality were reduced, but the intervention group did have a reduced incidence of a combined outcome of cerebro- and cardiovascular events (12.2% v. 39.6%, p = 0.004). Methodologic details, including blinding of outcomes assessors and numbers of patients excluded, were not described.

*Mixed ICU populations*
Four recently completed trials including mixed MICU/SICU populations also consistently failed to demonstrate an overall mortality benefit of achieving normoglycemia using IIT. A recently published fair quality trial used a two-by-two factorial design to assess IIT as well as two different types of volume resuscitation in MICU patients with severe sepsis.(29) This multi-center study used the Leuven protocol and was stopped early because of an excess risk of severe hypoglycemia in the intervention group (17.0% v. 4.1%; RR 4.11, 95% CI 2.21 – 7.63), with many of the hypoglycemic events classified as life-threatening (Table 4). Hypoglycemia was independently associated with mortality (HR 3.31, 95% CI 2.23 – 4.90). There was no significant difference between the groups for the primary outcomes of death at 28 days and multi-organ failure.

Three of the trials have not yet been published, but each of the authors shared methodologic and outcome details complete enough to allow quality rating and inclusion in our quantitative and qualitative analyses.(26-28)  GLUCONTROL is a recently completed fair quality randomized, multi-center trial that has been submitted for publication.(28) Using a insulin infusion protocol similar to the Leuven protocol, the IIT group was targeted to 80-110 mg/dl, and the comparator group was targeted to a more moderate range of 140-180 mg/dl. The trial was stopped after enrolling 1101 of a planned 3500 patients because of an excess risk of hypoglycemia in the intervention group (14.5 v. 3.9%; RR 3.64, 95% CI 2.30 – 5.75).(28)   Of note, the median blood glucose achieved in the control group (134 mg/dL) was lower than that achieved in the control groups in any of the other trials, further reducing the power to detect a significant difference in outcome between the two groups..  The ICU mortality rate – the primary outcome – did not differ between the two groups, but one month mortality was nonsignificantly higher in the intervention group (24.5 v. 20.7%; RR 1.19, 95% CI 0.95 – 1.48).  There was no difference in patient-days on renal replacement therapy between the two groups (521 v. 526, p = NS).

Another fair-quality MICU/SICU trial also found no significant difference in hospital mortality after adjusting for differences in baseline characteristics, notably a significantly smaller proportion of diabetic patients in the IIT group (Hospital mortality:  27.1% versus 32.3%, p=0.19).(26) Hypoglycemia occurred more often in the intensive group (9.1/100 treatment days versus 0.9/100 treatment days, p<0.0001).  There was no difference between groups in any of the secondary outcomes, including hospital mortality, ICU or hospital length of stay, duration of mechanical ventilation, need for renal replacement therapy or PRBC transfusion.

Finally, a poor quality trial found in-hospital mortality was similar between the two groups (I v. C, 32.3 v. 39.5%, p = 0.28).(27)  Nearly 75% of patients admitted to the two ICUs were excluded, most because the length of stay was projected to be < 48 hours.  The incidence of hypoglycemia was higher in the intensive group:  6.7% versus 0.8%, p=0.02 by morning whole blood glucose measures, and 41.3% v. 7.6%, p < .0001 by bedside glucometer measures.  There were significantly more patients with liver disease in the control group which may have contributed to the higher hypoglycemia rates.

*Meta-analysis*

Our combined analysis of all seven ICU studies(16, 22, 24, 26-29) evaluating the use of intensive insulin therapy targeted to normoglycemia found the intervention had a neutral effect on short-term mortality (Figure 3, RR 0.90; 95% CI 0.78 – 1.03, $I^2$ 40.7%).  A sensitivity analysis including the study that evaluated a more moderate glucose target (110 – 140 mg/dL compared to 140 – 200 mg/dL) produced similar short-term mortality results (RR 0.92; 95% CI 0.80 – 1.05, $I^2$ 38.7%).

**Figure 3.** Individual and combined estimates of mortality in MICU/SICU studies comparing intensive insulin with conventional therapy

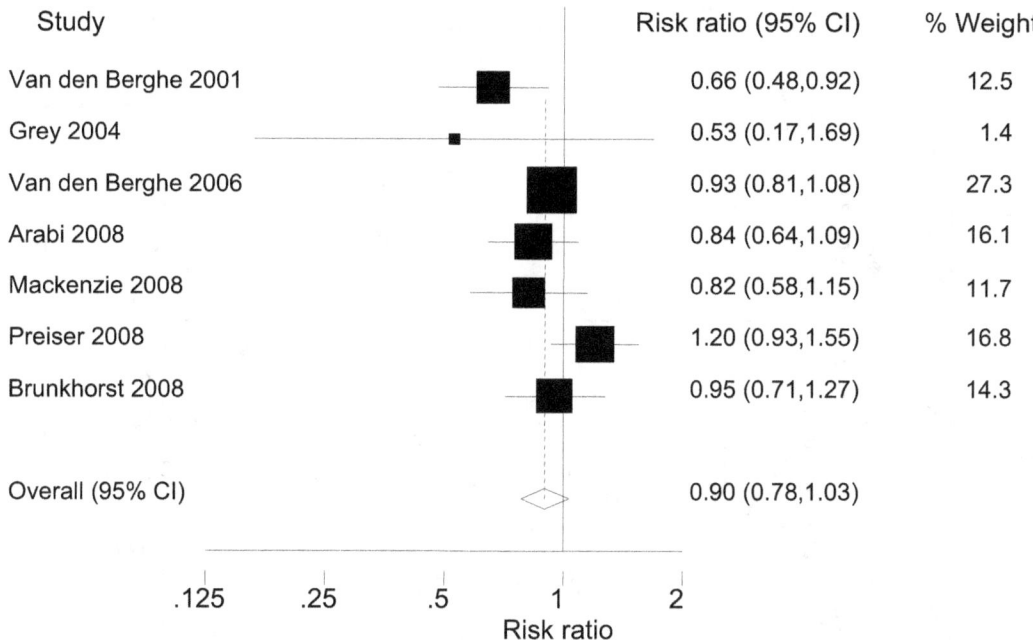

| Study | Risk ratio (95% CI) | % Weight |
|---|---|---|
| Van den Berghe 2001 | 0.66 (0.48,0.92) | 12.5 |
| Grey 2004 | 0.53 (0.17,1.69) | 1.4 |
| Van den Berghe 2006 | 0.93 (0.81,1.08) | 27.3 |
| Arabi 2008 | 0.84 (0.64,1.09) | 16.1 |
| Mackenzie 2008 | 0.82 (0.58,1.15) | 11.7 |
| Preiser 2008 | 1.20 (0.93,1.55) | 16.8 |
| Brunkhorst 2008 | 0.95 (0.71,1.27) | 14.3 |
| Overall (95% CI) | 0.90 (0.78,1.03) | |

Risk ratio

One good-quality meta-analysis of 29 trials evaluating tight glycemic control in critically ill patients was just published and similarly found no hospital mortality advantage (21.6 vs 23.3%; RR 0.93, 95% CI 0.85 – 1.03, $I^2$ 18%) or decrease in need for renal replacement therapy (11.2 vs 12.1%; RR 0.96, 95% CI 0.76 – 1.20, $I^2$ 25%) from IIT compared to usual care, but did find a reduced incidence of septicemia in the IIT group (10.9 vs 13.4%; RR 0.76, 95% CI 0.59 – 0.97, $I^2$ 35%).(43)  The authors included studies from a variety of settings which we considered separately, including neurologic, neurosurgical, and cardiac intensive care units.  They also combined trials which used different intervention group glucose targets:  a sensitivity analysis limited to trials achieving normoglycemia in the intervention groups found similar results.

*In-progress trials*

Several trials investigating the efficacy of achieving normoglycemia with IIT in critically ill patients are in progress.(33, 36, 37)  Of note, the NICE-SUGAR multi-center trial will be the largest to date and has randomized nearly 6000 medical and surgical ICU patients with results expected in early 2009.(33, 44)

# Table 1. Trials in patients in medical and surgical intensive care units

| Study | Population, Setting, N, % DM | Glucose target, T v. C (mg/dL) | Glucose monitoring method | Inpatient BG achieved, T v. C (mg/dL) | Mortality, T v. C (RR, 95% CI) | Concomittant therapy/nutrition | Quality¶‖ |
|---|---|---|---|---|---|---|---|
| (16) | SICU n=1548 13% DM | 80-110 v. 180-200 | Arterial blood samples | 103 v. 153* (p<0.001) | ICU mortality 4.6 v. 8% (p=0.005 unadjusted) RR 0.42 (95% CI 0.22-0.62); Hospital mortality: 7.2 v. 10.9% (p = 0.01) RR 0.66; 95% CI 0.48 – 0.92; New renal replacement: 4.8 v. 8.2% (p = 0.007) Sepsis: 4.2 vs 7.8% (p = 0.003) | On adm, all pts fed with IV glc; next day TPN, TPN and enteral, or enteral initiated; no sig diff between groups. 85.2 % received majority of calories through parenteral nutrition‖ | Fair |
| (24) | SICU n=61 15% DM | 80-120 v. 180-220 | Not reported | 125 v. 179† (p<0.001) | Hospital mortality: 11 v. 21% (p=0.50) RR 0.53; 95% CI 0.17 – 1.69 Sepsis: 4 fold increased risk of bloodstream infections in control group, numbers not provided | --- | Poor |
| (22) | MICU n=1200 16% DM | 80-110 180-200 | Arterial and capillary blood samples | 111 v. 153* (p<0.001) | ICU mortality: 24.2 v. 26.8% (p=0.31) Hospital mortality: 37.3 v. 40.0% (p = 0.33) RR 0.93; 95% CI 0.81 – 1.08 90 d mortality: 35.9 v. 37.7% (p=0.53) New renal replacement: 20.8 vs 22.7% (p = 0.5) | Mean kcal/d: Conv: 1238, Int 1202. 85.2 % received majority of calories through parenteral nutrition‖ | Fair |
| (23) | MICU, n=89 DM: 48.8% T, 68.8% C (p = NS) | 110-140 v. 140-200 | Not reported | 142 v. 174† (p<0.001) | ICU mortality: 39 v. 31.3% (NS) 28d mortality: 53.6 v. 45.8% (NS) RR 1.17; 95% CI 0.77 – 1.78 Sepsis: 26.8 vs 35.4% (p = NS) | --- | Poor |

| Study | Population, Setting, N, % DM | Glucose target, T v. C (mg/dL) | Glucose monitoring method | Inpatient BG achieved, T v. C (mg/dL) | Mortality, T v. C (RR, 95% CI) | Concomittant therapy/nutrition | Quality¶ |
|---|---|---|---|---|---|---|---|
| (29) | Septic patients in 18 MICUs, n=537 30% DM | 80-110 v. 180-200 | Arterial and capillary blood samples | 112 v. 151* (p<0.001) | 28 d mortality: 24.7 v. 26% (p=0.74) RR 0.95, 95% CI 0.70-1.28 90 day mortality: 39.7 v. 35.4% (p = 0.31) New renal replacement: 27.5 vs 22.5% (p = 0.19) | Mean daily caloric intake kcal/d 1236+/-534, p=0.47 | Fair |
| (28) | MICU/SICU n=1101 DM: 16.5% T, 21.8% C (p=0.031) | 80-110 v. 140-180 | Arterial and capillary blood samples | 108 v. 134* (p=nr) | ICU mortality: 16.7 v. 15.2% 28-day mortality: 24.5 v. 20.7%; RR 1.19; 95% CI 0.95 – 1.48 Days on renal replacement: 521 vs 526 (p = NS) | Percentage of days on parenteral nutrition: 26 +/- 44 % (T), 27 +/- 44% (C) | Fair |
| (26) | MICU/SICU N=523 DM: 32.0% T, 47.9% C (p = 0.0002) | 80-110 v. 180-200 | Arterial and capillary blood samples | 115 v. 171† (p<0.0001) | ICU mortality: 13.5 v. 17.1% (p=0.70) RR 1.09, 95% CI 0.70-1.72§ Hospital mortality: 27.1 v. 32.3% (p=0.19) RR 0.84; 95% CI 0.64 – 1.09§ New renal replacement: 11.7 v. 12.1% (p=0.89)§ | Mean daily caloric intake kcal/d 916+/-500 v. 830+/-509 >75% enteral | Fair |
| (27) | MICU/SICU - two centers n=240 14-19% DM | 72-108 180-198 | Whole blood monitoring | 126 v. 151* 113 v. 144‡ (p<0.0001) | ICU mortality: 19 v. 22.7% (p=0.53) Hospital mortality: 32.2 v. 39.5% (p=0.28) RR 0.82; 95% CI 0.58 – 1.15 | --- | Poor |

* Morning blood glucose

† Average of blood glucose measurements, not otherwise specified

‡ Time-weighted mean blood glucose

§ Adjusted for chronic liver disease, traumatic brain injury,APACHE II and INR.

‖Data from combined analysis of Van den Berghe SICU and MICU trials(45), data not reported in individual trials

¶The full quality rating for each study is provided in Appendix E.

## Acute Myocardial Infarction Patients

*Adjustable dose insulin infusions*

Six unblinded trials have examined tight glycemic control using adjustable dose insulin-based regimens (Table 2).(13, 46-50)  As a body of evidence, these studies lacked coherence and did not consistently demonstrate a benefit of adjustable dose insulin-based regimens in acute myocardial infarction patients.  Variation in trial design, achievement of recruitment goals, glucose level achieved, and concomitant therapy for myocardial infarction limit the strength of this conclusion.  (GRADE:  Low = Further research is very likely to have an important impact on our confidence in the estimate of effect and may change the estimate.)

Three trials of insulin-glucose infusions in patients with acute myocardial infarction had conflicting findings.(13, 46, 47)  The DIGAMI study was a fair quality trial,(13) in which intervention patients were maintained on an insulin infusion with the target plasma glucose 126 – 198 mg/dL for at least 24 hours and were subsequently transitioned to a multi-dose outpatient insulin regimen.  The control group did not routinely receive insulin.  Both groups were markedly hyperglycemic on admission (intervention mean 277 mg/dL, control mean 282 mg/dL, p = NS), but the intervention group achieved better in-hospital glucose control (172.8 mg/dL v. 210.6 mg/dL, p < .001) and maintained better glycemic control at one year of follow-up.  The three-month mortality rate did not differ significantly between groups, but the intervention group had lower mortality by one year (18.6% v. 26.1%, RR 0.69, 95% CI 0.49 – 0.96, p = .027).  It is unclear whether the benefit was related to the acute intervention or the longer-term insulin therapy.  Applicability of the study results to current MI populations may be limited:  only 50% of patients received revascularization therapy, the trial predates widespread statin use, and a large proportion (42 %) of eligible patients were excluded because of lack of willingness or ability to comply with a complex insulin regimen.

The DIGAMI II trial was a poor quality trial designed to determine whether the mortality benefit seen in the earlier trial was related to use of a tight glycemic control strategy during the acute hospital setting or the outpatient follow-up period.(47)  There were two intervention groups:  one received an insulin-glucose infusion and was transitioned to an insulin-based outpatient regimen, and the other received only the insulin-glucose infusion with subsequent diabetes care left to the discretion of the physician.  The trial was stopped early due to slow enrollment and the difference in blood glucose achieved at 24 hours between groups was smaller than anticipated (163.8 v. 180 mg/dL, p < .001).  Adjusted long-term mortality (mean follow-up 2.1 years) did not differ among the groups, though one analysis did suggest those treated with outpatient insulin during follow-up had a significantly higher risk of non-fatal myocardial infarction or stroke compared to those on oral glucose-lowering treatments (adjusted HR 1.71; 95% CI 1.25 – 2.35).(51)

A third fair quality trial investigated intensive insulin therapy given only during the acute post-infarct period with a moderate glucose target (72 – 180 mg/dL).(46)  The difference in blood glucose achieved during hospitalization between the two groups did not achieve significance (149.2 v. 162 mg/dL). There was no difference in inpatient, 3 month, or 6 month mortality between the intervention and control groups. Though there was a suggestion of reduced cardiac events and CHF in the intervention group, these reductions were not consistent across the follow-up period.

One small fair quality trial compared a normoglycemic to a moderate glucose target in survivors of ventricular fibrillation cardiac arrest.(48) Insulin infusion dosing was left to the discretion of the nurse without a strict protocol. The trial was stopped early after an interim analysis failed to provide any evidence of benefit. The authors found no difference in 30 day mortality, but the group randomized to a normoglycemic target did experience a higher incidence of moderate hypoglycemia (blood glucose < 54 mg/dL; 18% v. 2 %, p < .0001).

Two trials investigated the use of adjustable dose insulin as part of a glucose-insulin-potassium (GIK) infusion (Table 2).(49, 50) Van der Horst et al investigated a high-dose GIK infusion with a broad glucose target range in 940 patients with acute ST elevation myocardial infarction, approximately ten percent of whom had known diabetes.(49) There was no significant difference in blood glucose achieved between the two groups. There was no reduction in 30 day mortality in the overall group. The large prespecified subgroup of patients without signs of heart failure did experience a mortality benefit from GIK infusion (RR 0.28, 95% CI 0.1 - 0.75, ARR 3.0), but there were a large number of prespecified subgroups. A poor quality trial included a similar number of patients, with a similar proportion of diabetics, and found no difference in 30 day or one-year mortality rates between the two groups.(50, 52) The insulin infusion was targeted to a moderate glucose range, but the authors did not report blood glucose achieved or hypoglycemia rates in the two groups.

*Fixed dose insulin infusions*

We found good evidence that insulin used as part of a fixed-dose glucose-insulin-potassium infusion does not consistently improve final health outcomes in acute myocardial infarction patients, and may increase short-term mortality (not shown in table).(GRADE: High = Further research is unlikely to change out confidence on the estimate of effect.) An analysis combining results from two large fair-quality multi-center trials included nearly 23,000 patients and found no difference at 30 days in mortality (HR 1.04; 95% CI, 0.96 – 1.13; p = .33), development of congestive heart failure (HR 0.99; 95% CI, 0.93 – 1.06; p = .82), or reinfarction (HR 0.99; 95% CI, 0.84 – 1.17; p = .93).(53-55) Of note, in both trials the post-randomization glucose was higher in the GIK group, and the combined analysis showed an increase in 3 day mortality in the GIK group (HR 1.13; 95% CI, 1.02 - 1.26).

Three small trials of fixed high-dose GIK infusions reported clinical outcomes. One study of poor quality reported found no difference in mortality at 6 months.(56) Another fair-quality trial found a reduction in a composite outcome of short- (10.0 vs 32.5%, RR 0.24; 95% CI 0.09 – 0.63) and long-term (13.0 vs 40.0%, RR 0.22; 95% CI 0.09 – 0.55) cardiac events.(57) One small, poor quality study, hampered by poor reporting of follow-up, randomization, and allocation concealment, showed a reduction in congestive heart failure incidence.(58) Additionally, one fair-quality trial examined a fixed low-dose GIK infusion and found an excess in 35 day and 6 month mortality in the intervention group, with many of the excess deaths occurring within the first three days of the trial.(59)

One good-quality meta-analysis included 24 studies of insulin use in acute myocardial infarction patients.(60) The vast majority (n = 21) of these trials examined insulin in the form of fixed-dose GIK infusions, and 15 of these were conducted during the pre-thrombolytic era (pre-1990). When all studies, regardless of the form of insulin used or study date, were combined, there was a non-significant reduction in mortality (RR 0.89, 95% CI, 0.76 – 1.03). The pre-thrombolytic era studies seemed to account for most of this borderline benefit: when the 15 pre-thrombolytic era GIK studies were combined, there was a similar mortality reduction of borderline significance (RR 0.84, 95% CI, 0.71 – 1.00) while the six post-thrombolytic era trials found a neutral effect of GIK infusion on mortality (RR 1.02, 95% CI, 0.75 – 1.39). Three non-GIK trials included the two DIGAMI trials detailed above and a third smaller trial conducted prior to widespread thrombolytic use.(20) The authors could not pool these results because DIGAMI II did not report 30 day mortality outcomes.

## Acute Stroke Patients

There is very little fair or good-quality evidence investigating tight glycemic control in patients who have suffered a cerebrovascular accident (Table 2). (GRADE: Low – Further research is very likely to have an important impact on our confidence in the estimate of effect and may change the estimate.) The largest trial to date was poor quality and reported largely negative results.(61) The intervention group's glycemic target was very strict (72 – 126 mg/dL) while the control group only received insulin if blood glucose ranged above 300 mg/dL. The intervention group did achieve a lower 24 hour mean blood glucose (mean glucose difference 10.3 mg/dL; 95% CI 4.9 - 15.5), though this data was only available in half the population. The intervention did not reduce mortality or severe disability at 90 days. The trial was stopped early because of low participation rates.

A second much smaller fair-quality trial in patients with subarachnoid hemorrhage failed to find a long-term clinical benefit from tight glycemic control, but did find a reduced infection rate in the short-term (27% v. 42%, p < .001).(62) A small poor quality study included a subgroup of acute brain injury patients from a larger ICU trial.(63) Intervention patients received an insulin infusion but failed to achieve normoglycemic targets, and control patients received little insulin but received low glucose enteral feeds and intravenous fluids. There was no difference in ICU mortality or rates of neurologic recovery.

# Table 2. Trials in patients with acute MI or stroke

| Study | Population n % DM | Glucose target, T v. C (mg/dL) | Glucose monitoring method | Inpatient blood glucose achieved mean (SD), T v. C (mg/dL) | Mortality, T v. C (RR, 95% CI) | Concomittant therapy/nutrion, T v. C (%) | Quality * |
|---|---|---|---|---|---|---|---|
| *Insulin-glucose infusions* | | | | | | | |
| (46) | acute MI n = 240 DM 49% | T: 72 - 180 C: < 288 | capillary blood glucose | T: 149.4 (39.6) C: 162 (50.4) p = NS | Inpatient mortality: 4.8% v. 3.5%, p = .75 3 month mortality: 7.1% v. 4.4%, p = .42 | percutaneous coronary intervention: 32 v. 39; thrombolysis: 32 v. 32 most patient received aspirin, beta-blockers and statins (numbers NR) | Fair |
| (13) | acute MI n = 620 DM 39% | T: 126 - 198 C: NR | whole blood samples, bedside reflectance meter monitoring | 24 hours: T: 172.8 (59.4) C: 210.6 (73.8) p < .001 | 3 month mortality: 12.4% v. 15.6%, p = NS 1 year mortality: 18.6% v. 26.1%, RR 0.69; 95% CI 0.49 – 0.96 | thrombolytics - 50%, heparin - 17%, aspirin at d/c - 80%, beta blockers at d/c - 70%, insulin treatment at one year: 72% v. 49% (p < .0001) | Fair |
| (47) | acute MI, n = 1253 DM 77%* (with established DM, 23% had "newly diagnosed DM <1y) | group 1 and 2: 126 - 180 group 3: NR | NR | 24 hours: group 1: 163.8 (54.0), group 2: 163.8 (50.4), group 3: 180.0 (64.8) p = .0001 | Adjusted 2-year morality HR (95% CI): Group 1 v. group 3 = 1.19 (0.86 - 1.64) Group 2 v. group 3 = 1.23 (0.89 - 1.69) | percutaneous coronary intervention: 44 (gr 1) v. 40 (gr 2) v. 45 (gr 3) thrombolysis: 36 v. 34 v. 38 Aspirin at d/c: 89 v. 90 v. 84 Beta-blocker at d/c: 83 v. 84 v. 81 Lipid lowering at d/c: 67 v. 69 v. 57 | Poor |
| (48) | Ventricular fibrillation survivors n = 90 DM 11% | T: 72 – 108 C: 108 – 144 | arterial blood glucose | I = 90 (81 - 104.4) C = 115.2 (99 - 133.2), p < .0001 | 30 day mortality: 33% v. 35%, p = 0.85 | Therapeutic hypothermia | Fair |
| (63) | Acute brain injury N = 48 DM % NR 64.5% with CVA | T: 80 – 120 C: < 180 | Capillary blood glucose | Mean (inter-quartile range: T: 138.9 (125.6 - 174), C: 148.4 (131.5 - 188.6), p = .16 | ICU mortality: 25.8 v. 35.2, p = 0.5 | Enteral nutrition; control group enteral formula had lower % carbohydrates | Poor |

| Study | Population n % DM | Glucose target, T v. C (mg/dL) | Glucose monitoring method | Inpatient blood glucose achieved mean (SD), T v. C (mg/dL) | Mortality, T v. C (RR, 95% CI) | Concomittant therapy/nutrition, T v. C (%) | Quality |
|---|---|---|---|---|---|---|---|
| *Insulin-glucose infusions, continued* | | | | | | | |
| (61) | acute CVA n = 933 DM 17% | T: 72 - 126 C: < 306 | capillary blood glucose | 24 hour mean difference I v. C (95% CI): 10.3 (4.9 - 15.5), p < .0001 | 90 day mortality: 30.0% v. 27.3%, OR (95% CI) = 1.14 (0.86 - 1.51) 90 day severe disability: 35.1% v. 36.0%, OR (95% CI) = 0.96 (0.70 - 1.32) | NR | Poor |
| (62) | subarachnoid hemorrhage n = 78 DM 10% | T: 80 - 120 C: 80-220 | arterial blood glucose | NR | 6 month mortality: 15.0% v. 18.4%, p = NS Total infection rate: 27% v. 42%, p < .001 | Intracranial aneurysm clipping, intravenous calcium antagonists | Fair |
| *Adjustable GIK infusions* | | | | | | | |
| (49) | acute MI undergoing PTCA n = 940 DM 11% | T: 126 - 198 C: NR | whole blood samples | 16 hours: T: 138.6 C: 145.8 p = NS | 30 day mortality: 4.8 v. 5.8, RR 0.82; 95% CI 0.46 - 1.46 | Percutaneous coronary intervention: 91.6 v. 91.4 CABG: 4.0 v. 4.1 | Fair |
| (50) | acute MI n = 864 DM 10% | T: 108 - 180 C: NR | NR | NR | One year mortality: 5.3% v. 3.9%, p = .33 Recurrent MI: 4.6% v. 4.6%, p = .99 | Percutaneous coronary intervention: 94 v. 93 Thrombolysis: 1 v. 3 Aspirin at d/c: 95 v. 93 Beta-blocker at d/c: 91 v. 86 Statin at d/c: 88 v. 87 | Poor-fair |

*The full quality rating for each study is provided in Appendix E.

**Perioperative Patients**

Overall, the evidence, including five RCTs conducted in patients undergoing cardiac surgery,(64-68) is methodologically limited, evaluates heterogenous treatment approaches, and does not provide clear, consistent evidence of benefit from tight glycemic control strategies in the perioperative setting (Table 3). (GRADE: low = Further research is likely to have an important impact on our confidence in the estimate of effect and is likely to change the estimate.)

Two fair-quality trials were designed to evaluate the efficacy of achieving intraoperative normoglycemia using IIT during cardiopulmonary bypass.(65, 66) One trial which excluded diabetic patients found no significant differences between groups in rates of neurologic morbidity or mortality, but did find a trend toward increased hypoglycemia in the intervention group (11.7% v. 6.2%, p = 0.07).(65) In the second trial only the intervention group was targeted to normoglycemia during surgery, but both groups received insulin infusions with normoglycemic targets during the post-operative period.(66) More patients in the intensive insulin group than the control group died (2% v. 0%, p=0.06) or suffered a stroke (4% v. 1%, p=0.02) within 30 days after surgery.

Two RCTs examined the effect of GIK infusion administered just before surgery and maintained for 6-12 hours after surgery, using an adjustable-dose GIK infusion with a moderate glucose target range.(67, 68) One was a fair-quality trial (n=141) that found no significant differences in short-term mortality or MI, although GIK-treated patients had significantly higher cardiac indices (2.9 v. 2.4 L/min/m$^2$ after GIK infusion was discontinued at 18 h), less need for pacing (14% v. 39%, p=0.001), a lower incidence of infections (0 v. 13%, p=0.01), and shorter postoperative hospital stays (6.5 v. 9.2 days, p=0.003).(67) Survival at 2 years was marginally better among GIK patients in this study (p=0.04). The other study was a poor-quality pilot trial in 44 patients without diabetes, and found no differences between groups in wound infection, length of stay, or 30-day mortality.(68)

A poor-quality trial including CABG patients with diabetes (n=93) compared use of an insulin infusion to subcutaneous sliding scale insulin in order to achieve a moderate glucose target (150-200 mg/dL) in the immediate post-operative period.(64) The insulin infusion group achieved a lower post-operative mean blood glucose level (195 v. 288 mg/dL, p<0.001). There were no between-group differences in mortality, length of ICU stay, or frequency of sternal wound infections.

One good quality systematic review and meta-analysis included a large number of trials with patients receiving some form of insulin intraoperatively, perioperatively, and/or postoperatively.(69) The majority of trials included patients undergoing CABG, although a handful of trials examined other surgical populations. The authors included studies of GIK and insulin-alone infusions, and studies with and without a glucose target. Most trials were of poor to fair quality. We had excluded a number of these trials from our own review that did not examine prespecified health outcomes,(70-83) or that examined an insulin-based intervention without a glucose target.(70, 71, 73-76, 83, 84) When all

14 trials reporting mortality outcomes were combined, there was a 31% reduction in mortality (RR 0.69, 95% CI, 0.51 – 0.94).  However, when the Van den Berghe SICU trial(22) was excluded from the meta-analysis, the authors found no mortality difference between the two groups (RR 0.92, 95% CI, 0.57 – 1.48).  The Van den Berghe trial examined a qualitatively different intervention (ie – tight glycemic control throughout the ICU stay) and is extensively discussed along with the other trials examining glucose control in critically ill patients.

**Table 3. Trials in patients undergoing cardiac surgery**

| Study | Population Setting, N, % DM | Intervention and comparator | Glucose monitoring method | Glucose target, T v. C (mg/dL) | Inpatient BG achieved, T v. C (mg/dL) | Mortality, T v. C (% per group) | Concomittant therapy/nutrition | Quality * |
|---|---|---|---|---|---|---|---|---|
| (65) | CABG with CPB 0% DM n = 188 intensive IT; 193 saline placebo | T: Insulin infusion during surgery, if glucose > 100. C: saline placebo infusion. BG was measured for analysis. | Arterial blood samples | T: 70-100 C: not specified | T v. C levels were significantly lower (p<0.01), values not reported | In-hospital 2.1 v. 1.6% (p=ns) 6-month 3.2% v. 2.6% (p=ns) | 100-200 mL of dextrose 55 was administered when BG decreased to <70 mg/dl. | Fair |
| (66) | 48% CABG 52% other cardiac surgery 20% DM n = 188 intensive IT; 191 conventional IT | T: Insulin infusion during surgery, if glucose > 100. C: IV bolus of insulin if glucose >200; infusion if >250. Both groups received insulin infusion on arrival in ICU. | Arterial blood samples | T: 80 -100 C: <200 | After CPB, T v. C (mg/dL): 123 v. 148 (p=<.001) At arrival in ICU: 114 v. 157 (p<0.001) In ICU, both groups received IIT. After 24 hrs in ICU: 103 v. 104 mg/dL (p=0.72) | 30 days after surgery: 2 v. 0% (p=0.06) | During first 24 hr after surgery, pts were not given SQI or oral diabetic meds and received only clear liquids by mouth. | Fair |
| (67) | CABG 100% DM n = 72 GIK; 69 no-GIK | T: GIK infusion started just before surgery; continued 12h after arrival in ICU. C: SQ sliding scale insulin | Not reported | T: 126 - 200 C: <250 | 12 hours post surgery mean (SD) in mg/dL: T = 134.3 (3.7) C = 266.8 (6.3) | 30 days: 0 v. 0% 2 yrs: 0 v. 10% (p=0.04) | None. Pts resumed preop diabetic regimens (oral agents or insulin) after the 18-hr study period | Fair |
| (68) | CABG 0%DM n= 22 GIK; 22 D5W | T: GIK infusion started just before surgery; continued until 6h after reperfusion C: D5W placebo infusion, with no glucose monitoring | Serum | T: 89-179 C: not specified | NR | No deaths occurred within 30 days in either group | --- | Poor |

21

| Study | Population Setting, N, % DM | Intervention and comparator | Glucose monitoring method | Glucose target, T v. C (mg/dL) | Inpatient BG achieved, T v. C (mg/dL) | Mortality, T v. C (% per group) | Concomittant therapy/nutrition | Comments |
|---|---|---|---|---|---|---|---|---|
| (64) | CABG 100% DM n = 51 CII; 42 SQI | CII v. SQI. | Not reported | T: 150 - 200 C: 150 - 200 | Post-op day 1 mean in mg/dL (SD NR): I = 195.0, C = 229.1, p <.001 | Mortality: 3.9 v. 2.4% (p = ns) | Most patients returned to oral feeding during the 1st or 2nd postoperative day. Intermittent insulin injections were given instead of a continuous infusion once patients began eating. | Poor |

*The full quality rating for each study is provided in Appendix E.
Abbreviations: CII = Continuous insulin infusion; C = Comparator; DM = Diabetes mellitus; SQI = subcutaneous insulin; T = Treatment

## General Medicine Ward Patients

There were no studies evaluating a tight glycemic control strategy to less tight glycemic control in general medical ward patients.

*Observational Studies*

The following observational studies did not meet our initial inclusion criteria but we discuss them in further detail because they report health outcomes, have been cited frequently, and have informed clinical practice.

The Portland Diabetic Project was a single-center observational study of diabetic cardiac surgery patients treated between 1987 and 2005.(14, 15)  The control group consisted of patients treated between 1987-1991 during which time subcutaneous insulin was used to maintain blood glucose at or below 200 mg/dL.  An insulin infusion protocol was subsequently introduced in a graded fashion with glucose targets gradually lowered over time in an effort to improve staff/institutional acceptance and lower the risk of hypoglycemia.  Compared with the historic control group, the first intervention cohort, which was maintained on a peri- and postoperative insulin infusion with a moderate glucose target (150-200 mg/dL),  had a significantly lower risk of deep sternal wound infections (DSWI) (0.8% v. 2.0%, p = .01) even after controlling for patient level and surgical confounding variables.(17)  A subsequent analysis reported a lower cardiac mortality in the over 4500 patients enrolled during  the insulin infusion era compared with historic controls (1.1% v. 4.4%, p < .001).  The overall incidence of hypoglycemia was not reported.

In 2007 D'Alessandro et al used the EuroSCORE risk stratification algorithm to compare expected and observed mortality rates in diabetic patients undergoing cardiac surgery.(85-88) Between 2003 and 2004 patients were treated with an intra- and post-operative insulin infusion protocol similar to that of Furnary et al with target blood glucose 150-200mg/dL and a post-operative target of < 140 mg/dL.  Observed and expected mortalities in the historical controls were similar, while patients treated during the protocol era had a lower observed mortality than expected (OR 0.28; 95% CI, 0.09 – 0.82).  Morbidity rates, including DSWI, did not differ between the two groups.  The hypoglycemia rate was not reported.

Another observational study included mixed medical and surgical ICU patients admitted between 1999 and 2006 (89).  Mortality was compared before and after a protocol to maintain glucose between 80 and 140mg/dl was instituted in 2003.  The protocol prompted subcutaneous insulin use when blood glucose ranged 140-199 mg/dL and an insulin infusion when blood glucose exceeded 200mg/dL (the thresholds were lowered during the last year of the study).  The mean (SD) blood glucose was 124.4 mg/dL (51.3) and 154.0 mg/dL (87.5) in the post- and pre-protocol eras, respectively.  The authors found a lower mortality rate during the tight glycemic protocol era (OR 0.68; 95% CI 0.57-0.80, p<0.001) and most of this benefit was seen in nondiabetic patients.  The rate of severe hypoglycemia was relatively low overall, but increased during the protocol era (1.50 v. 2.26%, p = .051).

These studies have several important strengths: large size, consecutive enrollment, thorough follow-up, and an attempt to control for severity of illness and other confounding factors. They also provide important insights into the feasibility of establishing various glycemic control strategies in "real-world" settings. However, these studies also have several important weaknesses which temper their use in drawing conclusions about the efficacy of tight glycemic control in improving health outcomes and the use of specific glucose targets. Observational studies may overestimate magnitude of treatment effect when compared to randomized studies.(90) Because of the use of historic controls, it is difficult to ascertain the proportion of the health outcome improvement that was attributable to the insulin-based glycemic control strategies. For example, one study found a 25% drop in mortality within the subset of patients with the poorest glycemic control.(89) A number of interventions and quality improvement initiatives may contribute to improved outcomes in surgical and critically ill patients.(91, 92) The change efforts heralded by a glycemic control strategy may also improve provider and institutional acceptance of other quality improvement intitiatives and may reduce variation in practice around efforts such as infection control.(93) Also, as in the reviewed randomized trials, these single-center studies were necessarily unblinded and some improvement attributable to increased vigilance, more intensive training of staff, and more intensive data registry use is certainly possible. Finally, two of the studies did not report overall hypoglycemia rates, making it more difficult to draw conclusions about protocol safety.

## KEY QUESTION #2. What are the harms of strict blood glucose control in the above subpopulations?

The highest occurrence of hypoglycemia appeared among critically ill patients receiving IIT aimed at achieving normoglycemia (Figure 4, RR 5.32; 95% CI 4.21 – 6.73, $I^2$ 2.28%; Table 4), especially those in the MICU, of whom a large proportion had risk factors for hypoglycemia such as sepsis, malnutrition, liver disease, congestive heart failure, and renal insufficiency.(94-97)

**Figure 4.** Individual and combined estimates of hypoglycemia in MICU/SICU studies comparing intensive insulin with conventional therapy

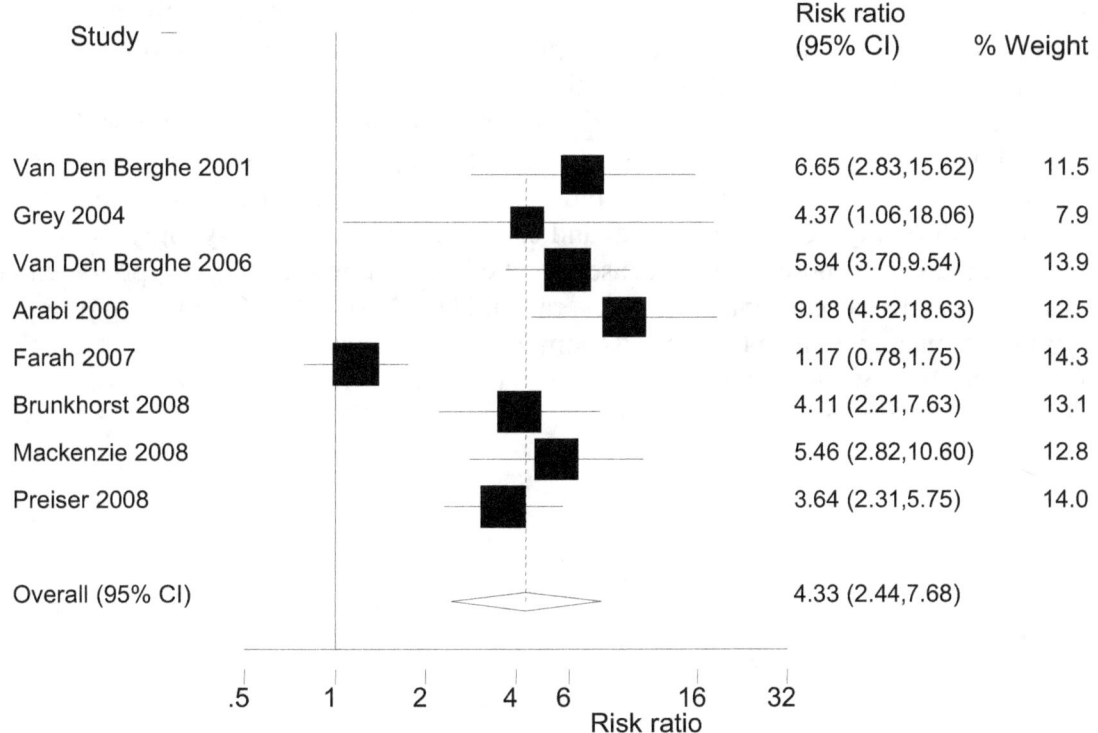

A recent fair quality meta-analysis included several of the same ICU trials(16, 22, 29) as well as several that did not prespecify health outcomes(98-101) and found a similar risk of hypoglycemia (RR 4.97; 95% CI, 3.65 – 6.76, p < .001).(102) Another recent good quality meta-analysis examined perioperative insulin infusions, many of which used higher glucose targets in the intervention groups: 20/34 included studies reporting hypoglycemia rates found that insulin-infusion was associated with a two-fold increased risk of hypoglycemia (RR 2.07, 95% CI, 1.29 – 3.32).(69)

The consequences of hypoglycemia in hospitalized patients are unclear. There were few reported in-hospital adverse effects of hypoglycemia during intensive insulin therapy in the reported RCTs (Table 4), though many critically ill patients included in these studies were sedated thus limiting the completeness of neurologic assessment. One study reported a case of cardiac asystole related to treatment-induced hypoglycemia.(103) Several MICU studies found an excess mortality risk or extended length of stay among patients experiencing one or more episodes of severe hypoglycemia, though it is unclear if hypoglycemia was a causative factor or simply a marker for more severe disease.(10, 26, 28, 29)

Most of the observational studies and trials without health outcomes that we examined used more conservative blood glucose targets and found far lower rates of hypoglycemia (Table 5). There was little information about hypoglycemia rates in general medical/surgical ward patients where staffing ratios, patient heterogeneity and diet may vary substantially.

Few studies have examined the long-term consequences of hypoglycemia. Svensson et al investigated the association between in-hospital hypoglycemia and 2 year all-cause mortality in a cohort of over 700 diabetic patients admitted with acute coronary syndrome. Hypoglycemia, defined as blood glucose < 55 mg/dL, occurred in 6.4% of patients and was associated with an almost 2-fold risk of 2 year all cause mortality (HR 1.93, 95% CI 1.18 – 3.17). Though comorbidities and other prognostic factors were controlled for, the study was observational and cannot explain whether hypoglycemia was simply a marker of more severe disease, or whether treatment-induced hypoglycemia itself can lead to adverse consequences. Several small studies(104-106) have suggested that hypoglycemia may induce transient ischemia and catecholamine surges, but these effects have not been well-studied in large groups of inpatients with the power to investigate downstream clinical consequences.

Table 4. Frequency of hypoglycemia in randomized controlled trials

| Study | Population | Intervention (T: treatment, C: control) | Glucose target (mg/dL) | Hypogly-cemia definition (mg/dL) | Frequency of hypoglycemia (% with one or more episode/persons studied) T v. C; Adverse events due to hypoglycemia |
|---|---|---|---|---|---|
| (22) | MICU | Insulin infusion in both groups*‡ | T: 80-110mg/dl C: 180-200mg/dl | <40 | 18.7% v. 3.1%;  AEs NR |
| (23) | MICU | Insulin infusion in both groups*‡ | T: 110-140 C: 140-200 | < 40 | Total # of hypoglycemic episodes per group:  23 v. 23;  AEs none |
| (29) | MICU | Insulin infusion in both groups*‡ | T: 80-110 C: 180-200 | <60 | 17% v. 4.1%, RR 4.11; 95% CI 2.21 – 7.63;  More episodes (T v. C) described as life-threatening (5.3 v. 2.1%, p = 0.05) and requiring prolonged hospitalization (2.4 v. 0.3%, p = 0.05) |
| (16) | SICU | Insulin infusion in both groups*‡ | T: 80-110mg/dl C: 180-200mg/dl | <40 | 5% v. 0.76%, RR 6.65; 95% CI 2.83 – 15.62;  AEs NR |
| (24) | SICU | Insulin infusion in both groups*‡ | T: 80-120mg/dl C: 180-220mg/dl | <60 | 32% v. 7.4%, RR 4.37; 95% CI 1.06 – 18.06;  AEs none |
| (26) | Mixed MICU/SICU | Insulin infusion in both groups*‡ | T: 80-110 C: 180-200 | < 40 | 28.6 v. 3.1, p < 0.0001;  ICU mortality in patients with hypoglycemia:  23.8% v.. 13.7%, P=0.02.  Among pts with hypoglycemia, higher mortality in IIT v. control group (25.0 v. 12.5%) |
| (27) | Mixed MICU/SICU | Insulin infusion in both groups*‡ | T: 72 – 108 C: <198 | < 40 | 41.3 v. 7.6%, p < 0.0001;  One case of cardiac asystole associated with rescue dextrose infusion in hypoglycemic patient |
| (28) | Mixed MICU/SICU | Insulin infusion in both groups*‡ | T: 80 – 110 C: 140 – 180 | < 40 | 14.5 v. 3.9%;  ICU mortality in patients with hypoglycemia: 32.2 v. 13.6% (p<.01) |
| (13) | Acute MI | T:  Insulin infusion*† for 24 hours then multidose insulin regimen for at least 3 months.  C:  usual care | T: 126 - 198 mg/dL C: not specified | <54 | 15.0 v. 0%, p < .001;  AEs NR |
| (46) | Acute MI | T:  insulin infusion* for 24 h. C:  usual care, supplemental insulin if glucose > 288 mg/dL | T: 72 - 180 mg/dL C: not specified | < 63 | 10.3 v. 1.8%, p = .02;  AEs NR |

| Study | Population | Intervention (T: treatment, C: control) | Glucose target (mg/dL) | Hypogly-cemia definition (mg/dL) | Frequency of hypoglycemia (% with one or more episode/persons studied) T v. C; Adverse events due to hypoglycemia |
|---|---|---|---|---|---|
| (47) | Acute MI | T: Int 1 - insulin infusion*† and outpatient multidose insulin, Int 2 - insulin infusion only. C: usual care | T: 126 - 180 mg/dL C: not specified | < 54 | Gr 1 v. Gr2 v. Gr3: 12.7 v 9.6 v 1.0; 1/3 of patients with hypoglycemia were symptomatic, no reported adverse clinical events |
| (50, 107) | Acute MI | T: adjustable high-dose GIK* C: usual care | T: 108 - 180 mg/dL C: not specified | NR | NR; AEs NR |
| (49) | Acute MI | T: adjustable high-dose GIK*† C: usual care | T: 128 - 198 mg/dL C: not specified | NR | 0 v. 0; AEs NR |
| (48) | Ventricular fibrillation survivors | Insulin infusion in both groups, no protocol | T: 72 – 108 C: 108 – 144 | < 54 | 18 vs 2; AEs NR |
| (61) | Stroke | T: Adjustable GIK infusion* C: saline infusion, insulin allowed if glucose > 306 mg/dL | T: 72 - 126 C: < 306 | < 72 for > 30 mins | 15.7, control group rate NR; AE s none |
| (63) | Acute brain injury | T: Insulin infusion‡ C: regular insulin if glucose >180 mg/dL; lower carbohydrate enteral formula | T: 80 – 120 C: < 180 | < 40 | 6.4 vs 5.8; AEs NR |
| (62) | Neurosurgical ICU, subarachnoid hemorrhage | Insulin infusion in both groups | T: 80- 120 C: 80-220 | NR | NR; AEs NR |
| (64) | Perioperative, CABG | T: Insulin infusion*† C: subcutaneous insulin | T: 150 - 200 C: 150 - 200 | NR | NR |
| (65) | Perioperative, CABG | T: Intra-operative insulin infusion* C: saline infusion. | T: 70-100 C: not specified | <70 | 11.7% v. 6.2% (p=0.07); AEs NR |

| Study | Population | Intervention (T: treatment, C: control) | Glucose target (mg/dL) | Hypogly-cemia definition (mg/dL) | Frequency of hypoglycemia (% with one or more episode/persons studied) T v. C; Adverse events due to hypoglycemia |
|---|---|---|---|---|---|
| (66) | Perioperative, cardiac surgery | T: Intra-operative insulin infusion* C: IV bolus of insulin if BG >200; infusion if >250. Both groups received 24h postop insulin infusion in ICU | T: 80 -100 C: <200 | < 60 | 1% v. 1% (p=1.0); AEs NR |
| (67) | Perioperative, CABG | T: Intra- and 12h postoperative GIK infusion* C: SQ sliding scale insulin | T: 126 - 200 C: <250 | NR | NR; AEs NR |
| (68) | Perioperative, CABG | T: Intra- and 6h postoperative GIK infusion* C: D5W placebo infusion, with no glucose monitoring | T: 89-179 C: not specified | NR | NR; AEs NR |

*Insulin infusion rate was based on current blood glucose
†Rate of change in glucose level was also included in adjusting insulin infusion rate
‡Factors included in insulin infusion rate calculations not reported, or protocol allows for dosing based on provider discretion
§Excess risk of severe hyperglycemia (BG>350 mg/dL) occurred in intervention group
Abbreviations: AEs = adverse events; NR = not reported

# Table 5. Frequency of hypoglycemia in observational studies and trials not reporting health outcomes

| CT, HC, or Obs. Study | Population | Factors included in insulin infusion rate calculations | Glucose target (mg/dL) | Mean glucose achieved mg/dL (SD) | Hypoglycemia definition (mg/dL) | Frequency of hypoglycemia (% with 1+ episode/persons studied) | Comments |
|---|---|---|---|---|---|---|---|
| Obs. (108) | MICU/SICU (no cardiothoracic surgery) 49.5% DM n = 90 | Current glucose<br>Rate of change in glucose<br>Current insulin rate | 75-120 | 133.5 (43.9) | <40<br><60 | 0.09*<br>1.0* | All patients received continuous 10% dextrose solution. Mean BG achieved was higher than intended (133.6 mg/dL). All consecutive patients on protocol were included, but it is unclear how patients were chosen for protocol. |
| Obs. (109) | SICU (47% cardiothoracic surgery) 35.5% DM n = 276 | Current glucose<br>Rate of change in glucose | 80 – 110 | 135.3 (49.9) | <60 | 1.5* | Included only glucose management service consult patients. Protocol did not achieve goal (mean capillary glucose 135.3 (49.9) mg/dL). |
| Obs. (110) | CTICU (2 centers) 34.0% DM N = 118 | Current glucose<br>Rate of change in glucose<br>Current insulin rate | 100 – 139 | Non-DM patients: 120.0 (14.0)<br>DM patients: 122.0 (9.0) | < 60 | 0.2* | Overall mean glucose achieved not reported. 73% within 80 – 139 mg/dL range. |
| Obs. (89) | ICU (66% med, 28% surg, 6% trauma) 21.4% DM n=2699 | Current glucose | 80-140 | 124.4 (51.3) | <40<br><70 | 0.58*<br>1.78* | --- |
| Obs. (111) | Burn-Trauma ICU 33% DM N = 30 | Current glucose | < 120 | 115.9 – 119.5 | < 60 | 5.0 | All consecutive patients on protocol were included, but it is unclear how patients were chosen for protocol. |
| Obs. (112) | Trauma ICU % DM NR n = 24 | Current glucose<br>Rate of change in glucose<br>Current insulin rate<br>Estimated insulin sensitivity | < 110 | 118.9 (27.3) | <50<br><70 | 0<br>2.0* | All consecutive patients on protocol were included, but it is unclear how patients were chosen for protocol. |

| CT, HC, or Obs. Study | Population | Factors included in insulin infusion rate calculations | Glucose target (mg/dL) | Mean glucose achieved mg/dL (SD) | Hypoglycemia definition (mg/dL) | Frequency of hypoglycemia (% with 1+ episode/ persons studied) | Comments |
|---|---|---|---|---|---|---|---|
| CT (113) | Trauma ICU 8.6% DM N=243 | Computerized algorithm Current glucose Current insulin rate | 80-110 | 116.0 (37.0) | <40 | 7.8 | Computer algorithm was compared to paper-based protocol with which hypoglycemia rate was nonsignificantly higher (11%, p = 0.25) |
| HC (114) | MICU/SICU (5 ICUs across 2 centers) % DM NR n = 2398 | Computerized algorithm; current glucose; rate of change in glucose; Estimated insulin sensitivity | 80 – 110 | 106.5 (39.1) | < 50 < 70 | 0.4* 5.0* | Treating physicians referred patients for infusion protocol. Each patient's estimated insulin sensitivity was part of the titration algorithm. |
| HC (98) | MICU/SICU 32.0 % DM n = 44 | Current glucose Rate of change in glucose | 90-144 | 128.0 (32.0) | <40 <72 | 0.2* 3.8* | All consecutive patients on protocol were included, but it is unclear how patients were chosen for protocol. |
| HC (115) | CTICU 32.0 % DM N = 168 | Current glucose Current insulin rate Presence of diabetes or steroids | 80 - 150 | NR % glucose within range: 61 | < 40 < 65 | 7.1 16.7 | Patients received no enteral or parenteral nutrition for first 24 hours post-operatively |

*rate reported as # hypoglycemic occurences/# total glucose measurements
Abbreviations: CT = Controlled trial; HC = study using historical control; Obs = Observational study

**KEY QUESTION #3. What are the most effective and safest means of lowering blood glucose in hospitalized patients?**

*Insulin infusions*

We evaluated three recent fair-quality systematic reviews,(116-118) of studies evaluating the effects of different insulin infusion protocols (IIPs) on glycemic control. There were no completed studies directly comparing these protocols, though we found two in-progress comparative effectiveness trials.(34, 35) The protocols differed in terms of patient characteristics, target glucose ranges, the time required to achieve the target glucose, the incidence and definition of hypoglycemia, the rationale or algorithm used for adjusting the insulin rates, the methods used to assess effectiveness and the methods of glucose monitoring. One review stressed that, given this variety of factors, each institution should individualize its approach to protocol implementation based on its patient population as well as its institutional and provider resources.(116) Another review focusing on ICU protocols used computer simulations to model patterns of insulin administration and similarly concluded that the variability amongst protocols precludes dissemination of a single protocol.(118) The authors suggest the better protocols incorporate bolus insulin doses, account for the direction and rate of glucose change, and make allowances for "off-protocol" adjustments. A third review concludes protocols that incorporate factors such as the rate of glucose change, the current blood glucose and insulin rate may be more effective than simple sliding scale infusion protocols in lowering blood glucose while maintaining relatively low rates of hypoglycemia, though this conclusion is not based on direct comparisons of protocols.(117)

Protocols used in observational studies and trials not examining health outcomes that we assessed are summarized in Table 5.(89, 98, 108-111, 113-115, 119, 120) Protocols used in the efficacy trials varied across subpopulations as detailed in Tables 1, 2, and 3. In general, protocols that were successful in targeting normoglycemia were also associated with a substantially elevated risk of hypoglycemia (Table 4). One observational study found a computerized insulin infusion protocol which incorporated factors such as insulin sensitivity achieved its normoglycemic target with relatively low rates of hypoglycemia.(114)

*Subcutaneous insulin*

Subcutaneous sliding scale insulin (SSI) regimens have a number of theoretical disadvantages when used as the sole method for inpatient glycemic control and authors have called for a reduction in the widespread use of sliding scale subcutaneous insulin.(121) A limited body of small, mainly single-center controlled trials suggest subcutaneous sliding scale insulin regimens may be relatively ineffective in targeting lower blood glucose. A prospective, multi-center trial compared a basal bolus regimen with SSI in general medical ward patients with type 2 diabetes and found the basal-bolus regimen led to longer duration of time within the target glucose range, from 38% to 66%, with no differences in the incidence of hypoglycemia.(122) A trial in patients with a glucose of more than 144 mg/dl after Roux-en-Y gastric bypass randomized the subjects (n=81) to SSI or insulin glargine.(123)   Mean glucose was 154 versus 134 mg/dl in the SSRI and glargine groups, respectively, p<0.01.  Hypoglycemia defined as glucose <60mg/dl occurred in only 3 of the 926 readings (2 in glargine and 1 in SSI). A randomized controlled trial of 153 diabetic patients admitted to a family medicine service found that the addition of a subcutaneous sliding scale insulin regimen to routine diabetes medications (oral agents or scheduled insulin) led to no difference in the time spent in the hyper- or hypoglycemic range (124).  A second trial randomized 93 post-operative cardiac surgery patients to either an insulin infusion or to a subcutaneous sliding scale regimen.  Mean blood glucoses of less than 200mg/dl occurred in more often in the infusion group (28.6 to 64.7%, p<0.001). (64).

# SUMMARY AND DISCUSSION

Observational and biologic plausibility studies suggest an association between hyperglycemia and worsening health outcomes in hospitalized patients. However, trial evidence of the efficacy of tight, compared to less tight, glycemic control strategies using IIT in various inpatient subpopulations is limited. Current evidence does not conclusively support existing guideline recommendations to routinely maintain a blood glucose ≤ 110 mg/dL in ICU patients, and there is very little data on the health outcome benefits of achieving more moderate blood glucose control (eg – 110 – 180 mg/dL) compared to less strict targets in various inpatient subpopulations.(125)

Single-center evidence from one group of investigators had shown a mortality and morbidity benefit from IIT in subgroups of patients requiring prolonged ICU stays, (16, 22) while our meta-analysis of seven ICU studies showed that achieving normoglycemia using a relatively simple insulin infusion protocol had no effect on short-term mortality but did substantially increase the risk of hypoglycemia.

Several factors may account for the discrepancy in results between the Van den Berghe trials and data from other centers. The aggressive use of parenteral nutrition, especially in the SICU study showing benefit,(16) differs from practice in many centers.(126) Parenteral nutrition has been associated with hypertriglyceridemia, insulin resistance, increased infection rates and mortality, leading to speculation that the observed benefits of intensive insulin in this population actually reflect a reduction in harm from aggressive nutrition practices.(127-131) It is unclear whether the control group mortality rate in this study was higher than expected. The authors of the study have reported mortality rates lower than expected based on the EuroSCORE of the cardiac surgery patients, though a review of EuroSCORE performance characteristics found that scores in the range reported in the trial may underestimate mortality by almost 3 %.(85, 132) On the other hand, a post-hoc analysis using combined data from both the Van den Berghe SICU and MICU studies found a mortality benefit in subgroups receiving the highest and lowest amounts of parenteral glucose.(45)

The exclusive use of arterial blood sampling in the Van den Berghe SICU study also has implications for the applicability of results across diverse ICU settings since very few medical centers use arterial blood sampling to monitor glucose control. Capillary blood sampling is more commonly used and is less dependable in critically ill patients, due to a number of factors including vasopressor therapy, perfusion pressure, pH, and others.(133-135) There is a very low rate of agreement between capillary and whole blood glucose samples, particularly in the hypoglycemic range.(99, 136)

Finally, this SICU study had a relatively low event rate and was stopped early for benefit with less than half the projected number of participants recruited, raising the possibility that the reported treatment effect was larger than the "true" treatment effect.(137) Indeed, the effect size decreased substantially, though remained significant, after the authors adjusted for the repeated interim analyses which had prompted the early recruitment discontinuation.(138)

Three of the trials that failed to show a mortality benefit from achieving normoglycemia in critically ill patients were stopped early due to an excess risk of hypoglycemia in the intervention groups, thus raising the possibility that the lack of observed benefit may actually reflect inadequate power to detect a health benefit.(26, 28, 29) However, the trials did not demonstrate a consistent trend towards benefit and combining these studies in our meta-analysis should increase the power to detect a health benefit if one were present. Furthermore, the inability to implement the insulin infusion protocol in various settings without high rates of hypoglycemia may underscore problems with feasibility and generalizability across institutions. It is unclear whether the high hypoglycemia rates are due to insulin infusion protocol characteristics, staffing characteristics, patient comorbidities, or the very tight glucose target itself. Since the health consequences of insulin-induced hypoglycemia in hospitalized patients are as yet unclear, interventions associated with high rates of hypoglycemia should demonstrate compelling benefit across a variety of institutions before being widely implemented.

The current body of trial evidence in perioperative patients is heterogenous and inconclusive. The most dramatic evidence of health outcome benefits from tight glycemic control in the perioperative setting comes from retrospectively controlled observational studies with methodologic flaws.(14, 15, 88) Well-designed controlled clinical trials in this population would add substantially to our body of knowledge.

Evidence supporting the efficacy of tight glycemic control in myocardial infarction populations is similarly limited and inconsistent. One trial showed a mortality reduction from moderate inpatient and outpatient glucose control in severely hyperglycemic myocardial infarction patients, but this older trial was conducted prior to the widespread use of cholesterol lowering therapies and mechanical revascularization techniques.(13) More recent studies have been negative, but methodologic considerations limit the strength of conclusions drawn from these trials.(46, 47) There is very little fair-good quality empiric data in general surgical or medical ward settings, or in stroke patients.

The ability to achieve glucose targets safely is likely to depend on multiple factors including the titration characteristics of the protocol, patient characteristics, as well as staffing ratios and provider acceptance. A number of mainly single-center observational studies and trials that did not examine health outcomes found relatively low rates of hypoglycemia. Characteristics of these studies suggest there may be several variables responsible for the lower rates of hypoglycemia: modest glucose targets (approximately 100 – 180 mg/dL), an iterative, institution-based protocol development and deployment process, and insulin protocol titration innovations. There is relatively little information on insulin protocols that have achieved normoglycemic targets with low rates of hypoglycemia.

## Limitations

Our review has several potential limitations. We did not exclude individual trials based on quality rating alone. Thus the strength of our conclusions is inherently limited by the quality variation among included studies. We did make an effort to note particular methodologic limitations, and each study was closely reviewed for overall quality using a rigorously developed approach. The studies included in our quantitative synthesis differed in some important respects: population studied and the attendant differences in event rates (ie – SICU v. MICU), interval of outcome reporting, and glucose monitoring method. The applicability of results from the included studies is limited by a variety of factors: patient characteristics, event rates, concomitant therapy, institution characteristics, and monitoring methodology. Most of these were single-center studies, yet the relative success or failure of an insulin-based intervention is likely to depend, to a significant extent, on systems characteristics which are unique to a given institution or health system. Finally, the included trials relied on glucose measurements from a defined reference time, rather than 24 hour glucose levels achieved, thus potentially obscuring the inherent variability in glucose control through the course of intensive care.(139)

## Future research recommendations

The bulk of efficacy evidence comes from studies in critically ill populations. Even amongst these studies, the patient characteristics, underlying event rates, and risk of hypoglycemia varied substantially. There is almost no empiric data available to guide glucose management practice in non-ICU settings. Future trials should enroll general medical and surgical ward patients.

The current body of evidence has not defined a glucose threshold that should prompt more aggressive intervention in various subpopulations. Given the observed risk of hypoglycemia in patients exposed to insulin therapy designed to normalize blood glucose, and the relatively low hypoglycemia rates in observational studies using less strict targets, the efficacy of higher glucose targets should be examined prospectively in various subpopulations.

As discussed, there are a variety of insulin titration protocols. Those that take into account a patient's insulin sensitivity and rate of glucose change are theoretically attractive, but future studies should rigorously evaluate these protocols and compare them to simpler protocols.

Individual institutions describing their experience implementing intensive insulin protocols suggest that the increase in nursing workload and fear of hypoglycemia were significant, but surmountable, barriers to implementation.(140, 141) The cost of attaining normal blood glucose in critically ill patients is unclear. Van der Berghe et al found that IIT targeted to normoglycemia was cost-saving using data from their SICU study.(142) Cost analyses using more recent data have not yet been conducted. Since insulin therapy can be resource intensive, future studies should examine the real cost and the opportunity cost of such treatment, as well as patient and staff acceptance across a variety of settings.

Transitions of care (e.g., ICU to ward, hospital to home) are fraught with uncertainty and there is likely a high rate of adverse events during these transitions, including an increased risk of post-discharge hypoglycemia.(143, 144) Studies should examine the safest and most effective ways to adapt insulin management in patients transitioning from one level of care to another.

There is a relative dearth of evidence evaluating the safety and efficacy of non-infusion based insulin protocols. Trials evaluating subcutaneous insulin protocols with moderate glucose targets in the medical ward setting would be of great use to clinicians.

Finally, newer technologies may enhance the safety and efficacy of inpatient glycemic management. Innovations such as continuous blood glucose monitoring systems and computer-based algorithms should be evaluated in various inpatient subpopulations.


# CONCLUSIONS

The use of intensive insulin therapy to achieve normoglycemia in critically ill patients does not clearly result in health outcome benefits and is associated with high rates of hypoglycemia. More moderate blood glucose control to targets above the normoglycemic range can likely be safely achieved, though the health outcome benefit of this practice has not been well studied. Tables 6 and 7 summarize the findings of this systematic review for each key question.

**Table 6. Summary of Systematic Evidence Review, Key Question 1: Does strict glycemic control compared to less strict glycemic control improve final health outcomes in the following patients?**

| Patient subgroup | Type of Evidence | Quality (GRADE) of Evidence | Comments | Net effect* |
|---|---|---|---|---|
| Acute myocardial infarction patients | 2 systematic reviews; 10 RCTs | High = Further research is unlikely to change our confidence on the estimate of effect. | We found good quality evidence that insulin used as part of a fixed-dose glucose-insulin-potassium infusion does not consistently improve final health outcomes in acute myocardial infarction patients, and may increase short-term mortality. | (−) |
| | | Low = Further research is very likely to have an important impact on our confidence in the estimate of effect and may change the estimate. | Several trials examined tight glycemic control using adjustable dose insulin-based regimens, and failed to demonstrate consistent evidence of benefit in acute myocardial infarction patients. Variation in trial design, achievement of recruitment goals, glucose level achieved, and concomitant therapy for myocardial infarction limit the strength of this conclusion. | (÷) |
| Acute stroke patients | 3 RCTs | Low = Further research is very likely to have an important impact on our confidence in the estimate of effect and may change the estimate | There is very little good-quality evidence investigating tight glycemic control in patients who have suffered a cerebrovascular accident. | (÷) |
| Patients in medical and/or surgical intensive care units | 8 RCTs | Moderate = Further research is likely to have an important impact on our confidence in the estimate of effect and may change the estimate. | Single-center evidence had initially shown a mortality and morbidity benefit from IIT in subgroups of patients requiring prolonged ICU stays, but the applicability of these data to other ICUs may be limited and subsequent trials have not confirmed this benefit. Our meta-analysis found the use of intensive insulin therapy to achieve normoglycemia had a neutral effect on short-term mortality, but increased the risk of hypoglycemia more than five-fold. | (÷) |

| Patient subgroup | Type of Evidence | Quality (GRADE) of Evidence | Comments | Net effect* |
|---|---|---|---|---|
| Perioperative patients | 1 systematic review, 5 RCTs | Low = Further research is likely to have an important impact on our confidence in the estimate of effect and is likely to change the estimate. | Overall, there is no clear evidence showing a benefit of tight glycemic control strategies in the perioperative setting, but the trial evidence is methodologically limited. The studies varied widely in design, blood glucose levels attained, and in the inclusion of patients with diabetes, limiting the comparability of results across studies. Several studies were underpowered to evaluate health outcomes. The best quality evidence of benefit comes from the single-center SICU study discussed in the ICU section. | (÷) |
| General medicine ward patients | None | Very Low = Any estimate of effect is very uncertain. | There were no studies evaluating a tight glycemic control strategy to less tight glycemic control in general medical ward patients. | (0) |

* (+) benefit; (–) harm; (÷) mixed findings/no effect; (0) no evidence

**Table 7. Summary of Systematic Evidence Review, Key Questions 2 and 3.**

| KQ# | Key question | Type of Evidence | Grade of Evidence | Comments |
|---|---|---|---|---|
| 2 | What are the harms of strict glycemic control in the above subpopulations? | 1 systematic review; 15 RCTs; 12 observational studies | Moderate = Further research is likely to have an important impact on our confidence in the estimate of effect and may change the estimate. | There is a considerable risk of hypoglycemia in medical ICU patients treated with intensive insulin protocols designed to normalize blood glucose. This risk was lower in surgical ICU patients receiving similar therapy, and in myocardial infarction, stroke, and perioperative patients in whom the target glucose level was generally not aimed at strict euglycemia. Observational studies suggest a moderate glycemic control can be safely achieved with modest glucose targets and variations in protocol design. Some studies suggest hypoglycemia in critically ill patients may be associated with excess mortality risk. The short-term and long-term consequences of hypoglycemia have not been well-studied. |
| 3 | What are the most effective and safest means of lowering blood glucose in the above subpopulations? | 2 systematic reviews; 2 RCTs | Low = Further research is likely to have an important impact on our confidence in the estimate of effect and is likely to change the estimate. | A number of insulin infusion protocols (IIPs) have been evaluated, but comparative effectiveness data are lacking. Protocols with moderate glucose targets appeared most feasible and were associated with the lowest hypoglycemia risk. Dynamic protocols that take into consideration the patient's insulin sensitivity and that have guidelines built into them to help prevent hypoglycemia may be preferred. The safe and effective introduction of insulin infusion protocols in a given institution is likely an iterative and multi-disciplinary endeavor. Basal bolus subcutaneous insulin regimens may be more effective than, and at least as safe as, sliding scale regimens, though there is very limited evidence comparing methods of blood glucose control in ward patients. |

# REFERENCES

1.      Atkins D, Best D, Briss PA, Eccles M, Falck-Ytter Y, Flottorp S, et al. Grading quality of evidence and strength of recommendations. BMJ 2004;328(7454):1490.
2.      Umpierrez GE, Isaacs SD, Bazargan N, You X, Thaler LM, Kitabchi AE. Hyperglycemia: an independent marker of in-hospital mortality in patients with undiagnosed diabetes. Journal of Clinical Endocrinology & Metabolism 2002;87(3):978-82.
3.      Levetan CS, Passaro M, Jablonski K, Kass M, Ratner RE. Unrecognized diabetes among hospitalized patients. Diabetes Care 1998;21(2):246-9.
4.      Furnary AP, Gao G, Grunkemeier GL, Wu Y, Zerr KJ, Bookin SO, et al. Continuous insulin infusion reduces mortality in patients with diabetes undergoing coronary artery bypass grafting. Journal of Thoracic & Cardiovascular Surgery 2003;125(5):1007-21.
5.      Pomposelli JJ, Baxter JK, 3rd, Babineau TJ, Pomfret EA, Driscoll DF, Forse RA, et al. Early postoperative glucose control predicts nosocomial infection rate in diabetic patients. Jpen: Journal of Parenteral & Enteral Nutrition 1998;22(2):77-81.
6.      Bochicchio GV, Salzano L, Joshi M, Bochicchio K, Scalea TM. Admission preoperative glucose is predictive of morbidity and mortality in trauma patients who require immediate operative intervention. American Surgeon 2005;71(2):171-4.
7.      Capes SE, Hunt D, Malmberg K, Gerstein HC. Stress hyperglycaemia and increased risk of death after myocardial infarction in patients with and without diabetes: a systematic overview. Lancet 2000;355(9206):773-8.
8.      Capes SE, Hunt D, Malmberg K, Pathak P, Gerstein HC. Stress hyperglycemia and prognosis of stroke in nondiabetic and diabetic patients: a systematic overview. Stroke 2001;32(10):2426-32.
9.      Rady MY, Johnson DJ, Patel BM, Larson JS, Helmers RA. Influence of individual characteristics on outcome of glycemic control in intensive care unit patients with or without diabetes mellitus. Mayo Clinic Proceedings 2005;80(12):1558-67.
10.     Krinsley JS, Krinsley JS. Association between hyperglycemia and increased hospital mortality in a heterogeneous population of critically ill patients. Mayo Clinic Proceedings 2003;78(12):1471-8.
11.     McCowen KC, Malhotra A, Bistrian BR. Stress-induced hyperglycemia. Critical Care Clinics 2001;17(1):107-24.
12.     Clement S, Braithwaite SS, Magee MF, Ahmann A, Smith EP, Schafer RG, et al. Management of diabetes and hyperglycemia in hospitals. Diabetes Care 2004;27(2):553-91.
13.     Malmberg K, Ryden L, Efendic S, Herlitz J, Nicol P, Waldenstrom A, et al. Randomized trial of insulin-glucose infusion followed by subcutaneous insulin treatment in diabetic patients with acute myocardial infarction (DIGAMI study): effects on mortality at 1 year. Journal of the American College of Cardiology 1995;26(1):57-65.
14.     Furnary AP, Cheek DB, Holmes SC, Howell WL, Kelly SP. Achieving tight glycemic control in the operating room: lessons learned from 12 years in the trenches of a paradigm shift in anesthetic care. Seminars in Thoracic & Cardiovascular Surgery 2006;18(4):339-45.

15. Zerr KJ, Furnary AP, Grunkemeier GL, Bookin S, Kanhere V, Starr A. Glucose control lowers the risk of wound infection in diabetics after open heart operations. Annals of Thoracic Surgery 1997;63(2):356-61.

16. van den Berghe G, Wouters P, Weekers F, Verwaest C, Bruyninckx F, Schetz M, et al. Intensive insulin therapy in the critically ill patients. New England Journal of Medicine 2001;345(19):1359-67.

17. Furnary AP, Zerr KJ, Grunkemeier GL, Starr A. Continuous intravenous insulin infusion reduces the incidence of deep sternal wound infection in diabetic patients after cardiac surgical procedures. Annals of Thoracic Surgery 1999;67(2):352-60; discussion 360-2.

18. van den Berghe G, Weekers F, Baxter RC, Wouters P, Iranmanesh A, Bouillon R, et al. Five-day pulsatile gonadotropin-releasing hormone administration unveils combined hypothalamic-pituitary-gonadal defects underlying profound hypoandrogenism in men with prolonged critical illness. Journal of Clinical Endocrinology & Metabolism 2001;86(7):3217-26.

19. Institute for Health Care Improvement. Establish a glycemic control policy in your ICU. In: http://www.ihi.org/IHI/Topics/CriticalCare/IntensiveCare/Changes/IndividualChanges/EstablishaGlycemicControlPolicyinYourICU.htm; 2008.

20. Davies RR, Newton RW, McNeill GP, Fisher BM, Kesson CM, Pearson D. Metabolic control in diabetic subjects following myocardial infarction: difficulties in improving blood glucose levels by intravenous insulin infusion. Scottish Medical Journal 1991;36(3):74-6.

21. Harris RP, Helfand M, Woolf SH, Lohr KN, Mulrow CD, Teutsch SM, et al. Current methods of the US Preventive Services Task Force. A review of the process. American Journal of Preventive Medicine 2001;30(3S):21-35.

22. Van den Berghe G, Wilmer A, Hermans G, Meersseman W, Wouters PJ, Milants I, et al. Intensive insulin therapy in the medical ICU. New England Journal of Medicine 2006;354(5):449-61.

23. Farah R, Samokhvalov A, Zviebel F, Makhoul N. Insulin therapy of hyperglycemia in intensive care. Israel Medical Association Journal: Imaj 2007;9(3):140-2.

24. Grey NJ, Perdrizet GA. Reduction of nosocomial infections in the surgical intensive-care unit by strict glycemic control. Endocrine Practice 2004;10 Suppl 2:46-52.

25. Mitchell I, Knight E, Gissane J, Tamhane R, Kolli R, Leditschke IA, et al. A phase II randomised controlled trial of intensive insulin therapy in general intensive care patients. Critical Care & Resuscitation 2006;8(4):289-93.

26. Arabi YM, Dabbagh OC, Tamim HM, Al-Shimemeri AA, Memish ZA, Haddad SH, et al. Intensive versus conventional Insulin therapy: a randomized controlled trial in medical and surgical critically ill patients. Accepted for publication.

27. Mackenzie IM, Blunt M, Ingle S, Palmer CR. GLYcaemic Control and Outcome in GENeral Intensive Care: The East Anglian GLYCOGENIC study. Unpublished report.

28. Preiser JC. NIH. Glucontrol Study: Comparing the Effects of Two Glucose Control Regimens by Insulin in Intensive Care Unit Patients. . http://www.clinicaltrials.gov/ct/gui/show/NCT00107601 Submitted for publication.

29.    Brunkhorst FM, Engel C, Bloos F, Meier-Hellmann A, Ragaller M, Weiler N, et al. Intensive Insulin Therapy and Pentastarch Resuscitation in Severe Sepsis. New England Journal of Medicine. 2008;358(2):125-139.

30.    DerSimonian R, Laird N. Meta-analysis in clinical trials. Controlled Clinical Trials 1986;7(3):177-88.

31.    Higgins JPT, Thompson SG, Deeks JJ, Altman DG. Measuring inconsistency in meta-analyses. BMJ 2003;327(7414):557-60.

32.    Egger M, Davey Smith G, Schneider M, Minder C. Bias in meta-analysis detected by a simple, graphical test. BMJ 1997;315(7109):629-34.

33.    Finfer S. NICE-SUGAR – A multi-centre, open label randomised stratified controlled trial of the effects of blood glucose management on 90-day all-cause mortality in a heterogeneous population of intensive care unit (ICU) patients http://www.controlled-trials.com/ISRCTN04968275.

34.    Iwamoto G. Comparative Trial Between 3 Types of Insulin Infusion Protocols clinicaltrials.gov, accessed 6/09/08;Study ID:NCT00582309; in progress.

35.    Umpierrez GE. Trial Between a Computer-Guided Insulin Infusion Protocol Versus a Standard Insulin Infusion Algorithm in Medical ICU. clinicaltrials.gov, accessed 6/09/08;Study ID:NCT00394524; in progress.

36.    Lacherade JC. Impact of 2 Blood Glucose Levels on Hospital Mortality in Patients Admitted in ICU (INSUREA). ClinicalTrials.gov;Study ID: NCT00591071; in progress.

37.    De La Rosa GD. Tight Glycemic Control in Critical Care Patients. ClinicalTrials.gov;Study ID: NCT00096421; completed.

38.    Azevedo JR, de Araujo LO, Azevedo RP, Silva WS, Cruz FL. Intensive insulin therapy versus glycemic control in critically ill patients: a prospective controlled trial. Critical Care 2007;11(Suppl 3):P82 (abstract number).

39.    Ingels C, Debaveye Y, Milants I, Buelens E, Peeraer A, Devriendt Y, et al. Strict blood glucose control with insulin during intensive care after cardiac surgery: impact on 4-years survival, dependency on medical care, and quality-of-life. European Heart Journal 2006;27(22):2716-24.

40.    Bistrian BR, McCowen KC. Nutritional and metabolic support in the adult intensive care unit: key controversies. Critical Care Medicine 2006;34(5):1525-31.

41.    Heyland DK, Dhaliwal R, Drover JW, Gramlich L, Dodek P, Canadian Critical Care Clinical Practice Guidelines C. Canadian clinical practice guidelines for nutrition support in mechanically ventilated, critically ill adult patients. Jpen: Journal of Parenteral & Enteral Nutrition 2003;27(5):355-73.

42.    Kanji S, Buffie J, Hutton B, Bunting PS, Singh A, McDonald K, et al. Reliability of point-of-care testing for glucose measurement in critically ill adults. Critical Care Medicine 2005;33(12):2778-85.

43.    Wiener RSMDMPH, Wiener DCMD, Larson RJMDMPH. Benefits and Risks of Tight Glucose Control in Critically Ill Adults: A Meta-analysis. JAMA 2008;300(8):933-944.

44.    Finfer S. In; Personal Communication.

45.    Van den Berghe G, Wilmer A, Milants I, Wouters PJ, Bouckaert B, Bruyninckx F, et al. Intensive insulin therapy in mixed medical/surgical intensive care units: benefit versus harm. Diabetes 2006;55(11):3151-9.

46.     Cheung NW, Wong VW, McLean M. The Hyperglycemia: Intensive Insulin Infusion in Infarction (HI-5) study: a randomized controlled trial of insulin infusion therapy for myocardial infarction. Diabetes Care 2006;29(4):765-70.

47.     Malmberg K, Ryden L, Wedel H, Birkeland K, Bootsma A, Dickstein K, et al. Intense metabolic control by means of insulin in patients with diabetes mellitus and acute myocardial infarction (DIGAMI 2): effects on mortality and morbidity. European Heart Journal 2005;26(7):650-61.

48.     Oksanen T, Skrifvars MB, Varpula T, Kuitunen A, Pettila V, Nurmi J, et al. Strict versus moderate glucose control after resuscitation from ventricular fibrillation. Intensive Care Medicine 2007;33(12):2093-100.

49.     van der Horst ICC, Zijlstra F, van't Hof AWJ, Doggen CJM, de Boer M-J, Suryapranata H, et al. Glucose-insulin-potassium infusion inpatients treated with primary angioplasty for acute myocardial infarction: the glucose-insulin-potassium study: a randomized trial. Journal of the American College of Cardiology 2003;42(5):784-91.

50.     Rasoul S, Ottervanger JP, Timmer JR, Svilaas T, Henriques JPS, Dambrink J-HE, et al. One year outcomes after glucose-insulin-potassium in ST elevation myocardial infarction. The Glucose-insulin-potassium study II. International Journal of Cardiology 2007;122(1):52-5.

51.     Mellbin LG, Malmberg K, Norhammar A, Wedel H, Ryden L, Investigators D. The impact of glucose lowering treatment on long-term prognosis in patients with type 2 diabetes and myocardial infarction: a report from the DIGAMI 2 trial. European Heart Journal 2008;29(2):166-76.

52.     Timmer JR, Svilaas T, Ottervanger JP, Henriques JPS, Dambrink J-HE, van den Broek SAJ, et al. Glucose-insulin-potassium infusion in patients with acute myocardial infarction without signs of heart failure: the Glucose-Insulin-Potassium Study (GIPS)-II. Journal of the American College of Cardiology 2006;47(8):1730-1.

53.     Mehta SR, Yusuf S, Diaz R, Zhu J, Pais P, Xavier D, et al. Effect of glucose-insulin-potassium infusion on mortality in patients with acute ST-segment elevation myocardial infarction: the CREATE-ECLA randomized controlled trial. JAMA 2005;293(4):437-46.

54.     Yusuf S, Mehta SR, Diaz R, Paolasso E, Pais P, Xavier D, et al. Challenges in the conduct of large simple trials of important generic questions in resource-poor settings: the CREATE and ECLA trial program evaluating GIK (glucose, insulin and potassium) and low-molecular-weight heparin in acute myocardial infarction. American Heart Journal 2004;148(6):1068-78.

55.     Diaz R, Goyal A, Mehta SR, Afzal R, Xavier D, Pais P, et al. Glucose-insulin-potassium therapy in patients with ST-segment elevation myocardial infarction. JAMA 2007;298(20):2399-405.

56.     Pache J, Kastrati A, Mehilli J, Bollwein H, Ndrepepa G, Schuhlen H, et al. A randomized evaluation of the effects of glucose-insulin-potassium infusion on myocardial salvage in patients with acute myocardial infarction treated with reperfusion therapy. American Heart Journal 2004;148(1):e3.

57.     Krljanac G, Vasiljevi Z, Radovanovi M, Stankovi G, Mili N, Stefanovi B, et al. Effects of glucose-insulin-potassium infusion on ST-elevation myocardial infarction in patients treated with thrombolytic therapy. American Journal of Cardiology 2005;96(8):1053-8.

58.     Turel B, Gemici K, Baran I, Yeilbursa D, Gullulu S, Aydinlar A, et al. Effects of glucose-insulin-potassium solution added to reperfusion treatment in acute myocardial infarction. Anadolu Kardiyoloji Dergisi 2005;5(2):90-4.

59.     Ceremuzyski L, Budaj A, Czepiel A, Burzykowski T, Achremczyk P, Smielak-Korombel W, et al. Low-dose glucose-insulin-potassium is ineffective in acute myocardial infarction: results of a randomized multicenter Pol-GIK trial. Cardiovascular Drugs & Therapy 1999;13(3):191-200.

60.     Pittas AG, Siegel RD, Lau J. Insulin therapy and in-hospital mortality in critically ill patients: systematic review and meta-analysis of randomized controlled trials. Jpen: Journal of Parenteral & Enteral Nutrition 2006;30(2):164-72.

61.     Gray CS, Hildreth AJ, Sandercock PA, O'Connell JE, Johnston DE, Cartlidge NEF, et al. Glucose-potassium-insulin infusions in the management of post-stroke hyperglycaemia: the UK Glucose Insulin in Stroke Trial (GIST-UK). Lancet Neurology 2007;6(5):397-406.

62.     Bilotta F, Spinelli A, Giovannini F, Doronzio A, Delfini R, Rosa G. The effect of intensive insulin therapy on infection rate, vasospasm, neurologic outcome, and mortality in neurointensive care unit after intracranial aneurysm clipping in patients with acute subarachnoid hemorrhage: a randomized prospective pilot trial. Journal of Neurosurgical Anesthesiology 2007;19(3):156-60.

63.     Azevedo JRAd, Lima ERM, Cossetti RJD, Azevedo RPd. Intensive insulin therapy versus conventional glycemic control in patients with acute neurological injury: a prospective controlled trial. Arquivos de Neuro-Psiquiatria 2007;65(3B):733-8.

64.     Li J-Y, Sun S, Wu S-J. Continuous insulin infusion improves postoperative glucose control in patients with diabetes mellitus undergoing coronary artery bypass surgery. Texas Heart Institute Journal 2006;33(4):445-51.

65.     Butterworth J, Wagenknecht LE, Legault C, Zaccaro DJ, Kon ND, Hammon JW, Jr., et al. Attempted control of hyperglycemia during cardiopulmonary bypass fails to improve neurologic or neurobehavioral outcomes in patients without diabetes mellitus undergoing coronary artery bypass grafting. Journal of Thoracic & Cardiovascular Surgery 2005;130(5):1319.

66.     Gandhi GY, Nuttall GA, Abel MD, Mullany CJ, Schaff HV, O'Brien PC, et al. Intensive intraoperative insulin therapy versus conventional glucose management during cardiac surgery: a randomized trial. Annals of Internal Medicine 2007;146(4):233-43.

67.     Lazar HL, Chipkin SR, Fitzgerald CA, Bao Y, Cabral H, Apstein CS. Tight glycemic control in diabetic coronary artery bypass graft patients improves perioperative outcomes and decreases recurrent ischemic events. Circulation 2004;109(12):1497-502.

68.     Smith A, Grattan A, Harper M, Royston D, Riedel BJCJ. Coronary revascularization: a procedure in transition from on-pump to off-pump? The role of glucose-insulin-potassium revisited in a randomized, placebo-controlled study. Journal of Cardiothoracic & Vascular Anesthesia 2002;16(4):413-20.

69.     Gandhi GY, Murad MH, Flynn DN, Erwin PJ, Cavalcante AB, Bay Nielsen H, et al. Effect of perioperative insulin infusion on surgical morbidity and mortality: systematic review and meta-analysis of randomized trials. Mayo Clinic Proceedings 2008;83(4):418-30.

70.     Boldt J, Knothe C, Zickmann B, Dunnes S, Dapper F, Hempelmann G. Influence of different glucose-insulin-potassium regimes on glucose homeostasis and hormonal response in cardiac surgery patients. Anesthesia & Analgesia 1993;76(2):233-8.

71.     Brodin LA, Dahlgren G, Ekestrom S, Settergren G, Ohqvist G. Influence of glucose-insulin-potassium on left ventricular function during coronary artery bypass grafting. Scandinavian Journal of Thoracic & Cardiovascular Surgery 1993;27(1):27-34.

72.     Koskenkari JK, Kaukoranta PK, Kiviluoma KT, Raatikainen MJP, Ohtonen PP, Ala-Kokko TI. Metabolic and hemodynamic effects of high-dose insulin treatment in aortic valve and coronary surgery. Annals of Thoracic Surgery 2005;80(2):511-7.

73.     Lindholm L, Bengtsson A, Hansdottir V, Westerlind A, Jeppsson A. Insulin (GIK) improves central mixed and hepatic venous oxygenation in clinical cardiac surgery. Scandinavian Cardiovascular Journal 2001;35(5):347-52.

74.     Lolley DM, Ray JF, 3rd, Myers WO, Sheldon G, Sautter RD. Reduction of intraoperative myocardial infarction by means of exogenous anaerobic substrate enhancement: prospective randomized study. Annals of Thoracic Surgery 1978;26(6):515-24.

75.     Oldfield GS, Commerford PJ, Opie LH. Effects of preoperative glucose-insulin-potassium on myocardial glycogen levels and on complications of mitral valve replacement. Journal of Thoracic & Cardiovascular Surgery 1986;91(6):874-8.

76.     Rao V, Borger MA, Weisel RD, Ivanov J, Christakis GT, Cohen G, et al. Insulin cardioplegia for elective coronary bypass surgery. Journal of Thoracic & Cardiovascular Surgery 2000;119(6):1176-84.

77.     Rassias AJ, Marrin CA, Arruda J, Whalen PK, Beach M, Yeager MP. Insulin infusion improves neutrophil function in diabetic cardiac surgery patients. Anesthesia & Analgesia 1999;88(5):1011-6.

78.     Rassias AJ, Givan AL, Marrin CA, Whalen K, Pahl J, Yeager MP, et al. Insulin increases neutrophil count and phagocytic capacity after cardiac surgery. Anesthesia & Analgesia 2002;94(5):1113-9.

79.     Raucoules-Aime M, Lugrin D, Boussofara M, Gastaud P, Dolisi C, Grimaud D. Intraoperative glycaemic control in non-insulin-dependent and insulin-dependent diabetes. British Journal of Anaesthesia 1994;73(4):443-9.

80.     Raucoules-Aime M, Ichai C, Roussel LJ, Romagnan MJ, Gastaud P, Dolisi C, et al. Comparison of two methods of i.v. insulin administration in the diabetic patient during the perioperative period. British Journal of Anaesthesia 1994;72(1):5-10.

81.     Wallin M, Barr G, oWall A, Lindahl SGe, Brismar K. The influence of glucose-insulin-potassium (GIK) on the GH/IGF-1/IGFBP-1 axis during elective coronary artery bypass surgery. Journal of Cardiothoracic & Vascular Anesthesia 2003;17(4):470-7.

82.     Visser L, Zuurbier CJ, Hoek FJ, Opmeer BC, de Jonge E, de Mol BAJM, et al. Glucose, insulin and potassium applied as perioperative hyperinsulinaemic normoglycaemic clamp: effects on inflammatory response during coronary artery surgery. British Journal of Anaesthesia 2005;95(4):448-57.

83.     Wistbacka JO, Lepojarvi MV, Karlqvist KE, Koistinen J, Kaukoranta PK, Nissinen J, et al. Amino acid-enriched glucose-insulin-potassium infusion improves hemodynamic function after coronary bypass surgery. A double-blind study in patients with unstable angina and/or compromised left ventricular function. Infusionstherapie und Transfusionsmedizin 1995;22(2):82-90.

84.     Valarini R, Sousa MF, Kalil R, Abumrad NN, Riella MC. Anabolic effects of insulin and amino acids in promoting nitrogen accretion in postoperative patients. Jpen: Journal of Parenteral & Enteral Nutrition 1994;18(3):214-8.

85.     Gogbashian A, Sedrakyan A, Treasure T. EuroSCORE: a systematic review of international performance. European Journal of Cardio-Thoracic Surgery 2004;25(5):695-700.

86.     Nilsson J, Algotsson L, Hoglund P, Luhrs C, Brandt J. Early mortality in coronary bypass surgery: the EuroSCORE versus The Society of Thoracic Surgeons risk algorithm. Annals of Thoracic Surgery 2004;77(4):1235-9; discussion 1239-40.

87.     Toumpoulis IK, Anagnostopoulos CE, Toumpoulis SK, DeRose JJ, Jr., Swistel DG. EuroSCORE predicts long-term mortality after heart valve surgery. Annals of Thoracic Surgery 2005;79(6):1902-8.

88.     D'Alessandro C, Leprince P, Golmard JL, Ouattara A, Aubert S, Pavie A, et al. Strict glycemic control reduces EuroSCORE expected mortality in diabetic patients undergoing myocardial revascularization. Journal of Thoracic & Cardiovascular Surgery 2007;134(1):29-37.

89.     Krinsley JS. Glycemic control, diabetic status, and mortality in a heterogeneous population of critically ill patients before and during the era of intensive glycemic management: six and one-half years experience at a university-affiliated community hospital. Seminars in Thoracic & Cardiovascular Surgery 2006;18(4):317-25.

90.     Ioannidis JP, Haidich AB, Pappa M, Pantazis N, Kokori SI, Tektonidou MG, et al. Comparison of evidence of treatment effects in randomized and nonrandomized studies. JAMA 2001;286(7):821-30.

91.     Hartl WH, Wolf H, Schneider CP, Kuchenhoff H, Jauch K-W. Secular trends in mortality associated with new therapeutic strategies in surgical critical illness. American Journal of Surgery 2007;194(4):535-41.

92.     Hedrick TL, Heckman JA, Smith RL, Sawyer RG, Friel CM, Foley EF. Efficacy of protocol implementation on incidence of wound infection in colorectal operations. Journal of the American College of Surgeons 2007;205(3):432-8.

93.     Haycock C, Laser C, Keuth J, Montefour K, Wilson M, Austin K, et al. Implementing evidence-based practice findings to decrease postoperative sternal wound infections following open heart surgery. Journal of Cardiovascular Nursing 2005;20(5):299-305.

94.     Fischer KF, Lees JA, Newman JH. Hypoglycemia in hospitalized patients. Causes and outcomes. New England Journal of Medicine 1986;315(20):1245-50.

95.     Shilo S, Berezovsky S, Friedlander Y, Sonnenblick M. Hypoglycemia in hospitalized nondiabetic older patients. Journal of the American Geriatrics Society 1998;46(8):978-82.

96.     Vriesendorp TM, van Santen S, DeVries JH, de Jonge E, Rosendaal FR, Schultz MJ, et al. Predisposing factors for hypoglycemia in the intensive care unit. Critical Care Medicine 2006;34(1):96-101.

97.     Krinsley J. Glycemic control in critically ill patients: Leuven and beyond. Chest 2007;132(1):1-2.

98.     Chant C, Wilson G, Friedrich JO. Validation of an insulin infusion nomogram for intensive glucose control in critically ill patients. Pharmacotherapy 2005;25(3):352-9.

99.     Kanji S, Singh A, Tierney M, Meggison H, McIntyre L, Hebert PC. Standardization of intravenous insulin therapy improves the efficiency and safety of blood glucose control in critically ill adults. Intensive Care Medicine 2004;30(5):804-10.

100.    Plank J, Blaha J, Cordingley J, Wilinska ME, Chassin LJ, Morgan C, et al. Multicentric, randomized, controlled trial to evaluate blood glucose control by the model predictive control algorithm versus routine glucose management protocols in intensive care unit patients. Diabetes Care 2006;29(2):271-6.

101.    Toft P, Jorgensen HS, Toennesen E, Christiansen C. Intensive insulin therapy to non-cardiac ICU patients: a prospective study. European Journal of Anaesthesiology 2006;23(8):705-9.

102.    Mechanick JI, Handelsman Y, Bloomgarden ZT. Hypoglycemia in the intensive care unit. Current Opinion in Clinical Nutrition & Metabolic Care 2007;10(2):193-6.

103.    Mackenzie I, Ingle S, Zaidi S, Buczaski S. Tight glycaemic control: a survey of intensive care practice in large English hospitals. Intensive Care Medicine 2005;31(8):1136.

104.    Desouza C, Salazar H, Cheong B, Murgo J, Fonseca V. Association of hypoglycemia and cardiac ischemia: a study based on continuous monitoring. Diabetes Care 2003;26(5):1485-9.

105.    Lindstrom T, Jorfeldt L, Tegler L, Arnqvist HJ. Hypoglycaemia and cardiac arrhythmias in patients with type 2 diabetes mellitus. Diabetic Medicine 1992;9(6):536-41.

106.    Spyer G, Hattersley AT, MacDonald IA, Amiel S, MacLeod KM. Hypoglycaemic counter-regulation at normal blood glucose concentrations in patients with well controlled type-2 diabetes. Lancet 2000;356(9246):1970-4.

107.    van der Horst ICC, De Luca G, Ottervanger JP, de Boer M-J, Hoorntje JCA, Suryapranata H, et al. ST-segment elevation resolution and outcome in patients treated with primary angioplasty and glucose-insulin-potassium infusion. American Heart Journal 2005;149(6):1135.

108.    Balkin M, Mascioli C, Smith V, Alnachawati H, Mehrishi S, Saydain G, et al. Achieving durable glucose control in the intensive care unit without hypoglycaemia: a new practical IV insulin protocol. Diabetes/Metabolism Research Reviews 2007;23(1):49-55.

109.    DeSantis AJ, Schmeltz LR, Schmidt K, O'Shea-Mahler E, Rhee C, Wells A, et al. Inpatient management of hyperglycemia: the Northwestern experience. Endocrine Practice 2006;12(5):491-505.

110.    Goldberg PA, Sakharova OV, Barrett PW, Falko LN, Roussel MG, Bak L, et al. Improving glycemic control in the cardiothoracic intensive care unit: clinical experience in two hospital settings. Journal of Cardiothoracic & Vascular Anesthesia 2004;18(6):690-7.

111.    Cochran A, Davis L, Morris SE, Saffle JR. Safety and efficacy of an intensive insulin protocol in a burn-trauma intensive care unit. Journal of Burn Care & Research 2008;29(1):187-91.

112.    Braithwaite SS, Edkins R, Macgregor KL, Sredzienski ES, Houston M, Zarzaur B, et al. Performance of a dose-defining insulin infusion protocol among trauma service intensive care unit admissions. Diabetes Technology & Therapeutics 2006;8(4):476-88.

113.    Dortch MJ, Mowery NT, Ozdas A, Dossett L, Cao H, Collier B, et al. A computerized insulin infusion titration protocol improves glucose control with less hypoglycemia compared to a manual titration protocol in a trauma intensive care unit. Jpen: Journal of Parenteral & Enteral Nutrition 2008;32(1):18-27.

114.    Juneja R, Roudebush C, Kumar N, Macy A, Golas A, Wall D, et al. Utilization of a computerized intravenous insulin infusion program to control blood glucose in the intensive care unit. Diabetes Technology & Therapeutics 2007;9(3):232-40.

115.    Zimmerman CR, Mlynarek ME, Jordan JA, Rajda CA, Horst HM. An insulin infusion protocol in critically ill cardiothoracic surgery patients. Annals of Pharmacotherapy 2004;38(7-8):1123-9.

116.    Nazer LH, Chow SL, Moghissi ES. Insulin infusion protocols for critically ill patients: a highlight of differences and similarities. Endocrine Practice 2007;13(2):137-46.

117.    Meijering S, Corstjens AM, Tulleken JE, Meertens JHJM, Zijlstra JG, Ligtenberg JJM. Towards a feasible algorithm for tight glycaemic control in critically ill patients: a systematic review of the literature. Critical Care (London, England) 2006;10(1):R19.

118.    Wilson M, Weinreb J, Hoo GW, Wilson M, Weinreb J, Hoo GWS. Intensive insulin therapy in critical care: a review of 12 protocols. Diabetes Care 2007;30(4):1005-11.

119.    Elinav H, Wolf Z, Szalat A, Bdolah-Abram T, Glaser B, Raz I, et al. In-hospital treatment of hyperglycemia: effects of intensified subcutaneous insulin treatment. Current Medical Research & Opinion 2007;23(4):757-65.

120.    Miriam A, Korula G. A simple glucose insulin regimen for perioperative blood glucose control: the Vellore regimen. Anesthesia & Analgesia 2004;99(2):598-602.

121.    Metchick LN, Petit WA, Jr., Inzucchi SE, Department of Medicine UoCSoMFC, Joslin Diabetes Center NBC, Section of Endocrinology DoMYUSoMNHC. Inpatient management of diabetes mellitus. American Journal of Medicine 2002;113(4):317-23.

122.    Umpierrez GE, Smiley D, Zisman A, Prieto LM, Palacio A, Ceron M, et al. Randomized study of basal-bolus insulin therapy in the inpatient management of patients with type 2 diabetes (RABBIT 2 trial). Diabetes Care 2007;30(9):2181-6.

123.    Datta S, Qaadir A, Villanueva G, Baldwin D. Once-daily insulin glargine versus 6-hour sliding scale regular insulin for control of hyperglycemia after a bariatric surgical procedure: a randomized clinical trial. Endocrine Practice 2007;13(3):225-31.

124.    Dickerson LM, Ye X, Sack JL, Hueston WJ. Glycemic control in medical inpatients with type 2 diabetes mellitus receiving sliding scale insulin regimens versus routine diabetes medications: a multicenter randomized controlled trial. Annals of Family Medicine 2003;1(1):29-35.

125.    Garber AJ, Moghissi ES, Bransome ED, Jr., Clark NG, Clement S, Cobin RH, et al. American College of Endocrinology position statement on inpatient diabetes and metabolic control. Endocrine Practice 2004;10(1):77-82.

126.    Needham PJ, Burton AB, Jayne DG. Artifical nutrition in UK intensive care units: a review of current practice. Proceedings of the Nutrition Society 2008;67((OCE)):E152.

127.    Lewis KS, Kane-Gill SL, Bobek MB, Dasta JF. Intensive insulin therapy for critically ill patients. Annals of Pharmacotherapy 2004;38(7-8):1243-51.

128.    O'Keefe SJD, Lee RB, Anderson FP, Gennings C, Abou-Assi S, Clore J, et al. Physiological effects of enteral and parenteral feeding on pancreaticobiliary secretion in

humans. American Journal of Physiology - Gastrointestinal & Liver Physiology 2003;284(1):G27-36.

129.    Braunschweig CL, Levy P, Sheean PM, Wang X. Enteral compared with parenteral nutrition: a meta-analysis. American Journal of Clinical Nutrition 2001;74(4):534-42.

130.    Klein CJ, Stanek GS, Wiles CE, 3rd. Overfeeding macronutrients to critically ill adults: metabolic complications. Journal of the American Dietetic Association 1998;98(7):795-806.

131.    Brunkhorst F, Reinhart K, Engel C. Insulin and Pentastarch for Severe Sepsis. New England Journal of Medicine 2008;358(19):2074-2075.

132.    Van den Berghe G, Wilmer A, Bouillon R, Van den Berghe G, Wilmer A, Bouillon R. Insulin and pentastarch for severe sepsis. New England Journal of Medicine 2008;358(19):2073; author reply 2074-5.

133.    Atkin SH, Dasmahapatra A, Jaker MA, Chorost MI, Reddy S. Fingerstick glucose determination in shock. Annals of Internal Medicine 1991;114(12):1020-4.

134.    Critchell CD, Savarese V, Callahan A, Aboud C, Jabbour S, Marik P. Accuracy of bedside capillary blood glucose measurements in critically ill patients. Intensive Care Medicine 2007;33(12):2079-84.

135.    Tanvetyanon T, Walkenstein MD, Marra A. Inaccurate glucose determination by fingerstick in a patient with peripheral arterial disease. Annals of Internal Medicine 2002;137(9):W1.

136.    Desachy A, Vuagnat AC, Ghazali AD, Baudin OT, Longuet OH, Calvat SN, et al. Accuracy of bedside glucometry in critically ill patients: influence of clinical characteristics and perfusion index. Mayo Clinic Proceedings 2008;83(4):400-5.

137.    Montori VM, Devereaux PJ, Adhikari NKJ, Burns KEA, Eggert CH, Briel M, et al. Randomized Trials Stopped Early for Benefit: A Systematic Review. JAMA 2005;294(17):2203-2209.

138.    Lan KKG, DeMets DL. Discrete sequential boundaries for clinical trials. Biometrika 1983;70(3):659-663.

139.    Finney SJ, Zekveld C, Elia A, Evans TW, Finney SJ, Zekveld C, et al. Glucose control and mortality in critically ill patients. JAMA 2003;290(15):2041-7.

140.    Goldberg PA, Inzucchi SE. Selling root canals:  lessons learned from implementing a hospital insulin infusion protocol. Diabetes Spectrum 2005;18(1):28-33.

141.    Rea RS, Donihi AC, Bobeck M, Herout P, McKaveney TP, Kane-Gill SL, et al. Implementing an intravenous insulin infusion protocol in the intensive care unit. American Journal of Health-System Pharmacy 2007;64(4):385-95.

142.    Van den Berghe G, Wouters PJ, Kesteloot K, Hilleman DE. Analysis of healthcare resource utilization with intensive insulin therapy in critically ill patients. Critical Care Medicine 2006;34(3):612-6.

143.    Forster AJ, Murff HJ, Peterson JF, Gandhi TK, Bates DW. The incidence and severity of adverse events affecting patients after discharge from the hospital. Annals of Internal Medicine 2003;138(3):161-7.

144.    Shorr RI, Ray WA, Daugherty JR, Griffin MR. Incidence and risk factors for serious hypoglycemia in older persons using insulin or sulfonylureas. Archives of Internal Medicine 1997;157(15):1681-6.

# APPENDIX A.  SEARCH STRATEGY

Database: Ovid MEDLINE(R) <1950 to November Week 2 2007>
Search Strategy:
--------------------------------------------------------------------------------
1    exp insulin/ (130835)
2    exp hypoglycemic agents/ (151706)
3    exp Blood Glucose/ (98489)
4    (insulin or hypoglycemic agent$ or hypoglycaemic agent$ or glycemic control or glycaemic control).mp. [mp=title, original title, abstract, name of substance word, subject heading word] (243159)
5    1 or 2 or 3 or 4 (292506)
6    Critical Illness/ (8301)
7    critical care/ or intensive care/ (28092)
8    exp Perioperative Care/ (60582)
9    exp Postoperative Period/ (28181)
10    ((critical$ adj6 ill$) or critical care or icu or intensive care or burn unit$ or coronary care).mp. [mp=title, original title, abstract, name of substance word, subject heading word] (103498)
11    intensive care units/ or burn units/ or coronary care units/ or recovery room/ (27247)
12    postoperative complications/ or prosthesis-related infections/ or surgical wound dehiscence/ or surgical wound infection/ (252519)
13    (postoperative$ or post operative$).mp. [mp=title, original title, abstract, name of substance word, subject heading word] (457854)
14    6 or 7 or 8 or 9 or 10 or 11 or 12 or 13 (582795)
15    5 and 14 (5822)
16    randomized controlled trial.pt. (246761)
17    controlled clinical trial.pt. (77022)
18    randomized controlled trials.sh. (52472)
19    random allocation.sh. (59778)
20    double blind method.sh. (94781)
21    single blind method.sh. (11591)
22    16 or 17 or 18 or 19 or 20 or 21 (418296)
23    (animals not human).sh. (4261058)
24    22 not 23 (382274)
25    clinical trial.pt. (444490)
26    exp clinical trials/ (199910)
27    (clin$ adj25 trial$).ti,ab. (139332)
28    ((singl$ or doubl$ or trebl$ or tripl$) adj25 (blind$ or mask$)).ti,ab. (94254)
29    placebos.sh. (26956)
30    placebo$.ti,ab. (106977)
31    random$.ti,ab. (394441)
32    research design.sh. (50582)
33    25 or 26 or 27 or 28 or 29 or 30 or 31 or 32 (887876)
34    33 not 23 (778635)

35  34 or 24 (798240)
36  15 and 35 (979)
37  exp Myocardial Infarction/ (115916)
38  exp Hospitalization/ (107713)
39  exp Inpatients/ (6673)
40  exp Cerebrovascular Accident/ (44100)
41  cerebrovascular disorders/ or brain ischemia/ or exp "intracranial embolism and thrombosis"/ or exp intracranial hemorrhages/ (112871)
42  exp myocardial revascularization/ or exp coronary artery bypass/ (56866)
43  37 or 40 or 41 or 42 (300510)
44  5 and 43 (4061)
45  35 and 44 (657)
46  45 not 36 (544)
47  38 or 39 (113294)
48  5 and 47 (1078)
49  35 and 48 (202)
50  49 not (36 or 46) (114)
51  exp Hypoglycemia/ci, ep, et [Chemically Induced, Epidemiology, Etiology] (8651)
52  1 or 2 or 4 (250082)
53  51 and 52 (5520)
54  14 and 53 (180)
55  43 and 53 (41)
56  47 and 53 (65)
57  54 or 55 or 56 (276)
58  57 not (36 or 46 or 49) (254)
59  exp Hypoglycemia/ (17277)
60  52 and 59 (9545)
61  14 and 60 (285)
62  43 and 60 (86)
63  47 and 60 (97)
64  61 or 62 or 63 (445)
65  64 not 57 (169)
66  65 not (36 or 46 or 49) (152)
67  limit 36 to english language (865)
68  limit 46 to english language (476)
69  limit 50 to english language (104)
70  limit 58 to english language (215)
71  limit 66 to english language (113)
72  from 67 keep 1-865 (865)
73  from 68 keep 1-476 (476)
74  from 69 keep 1-104 (104)
75  from 70 keep 1-215 (215)
76  from 71 keep 1-113 (113)


*************************

An additional search for adverse effects used the strategy above through line 71, followed by:

72    (ae or po or to).fs. (1254721)
73    exp Drug Toxicity/ (15829)
74    medical errors/ or medication errors/ (13158)
75    exp Drug Interactions/ (116890)
76    72 or 73 or 74 or 75 (1359022)
77    1 or 3 (186918)
78    6 or 7 or 8 or 9 or 11 or 12 (379861)
79    77 and 78 (2545)
80    76 and 79 (364)
81    limit 80 to english language (296)
82    limit 81 to humans (276)
83    15 and 76 (871)
84    limit 83 to english language (725)
85    limit 84 to humans (668)
86    85 not 82 (392)
87    from 82 keep 1-276 (276)
88    from 86 keep 1-392 (392)


*************************

# APPENDIX B.  INCLUSION/EXCLUSION CRITERIA

| Code | Include / Exclude | *Reason* |
|------|-------------------|----------|
| I | Include | Clinical trial, cohort study, systematic review/meta-analysis of studies that<br>  A.  Were conducted in any of the following populations:<br>    1. Acute myocardial infarction patients<br>    2. Other patients in the medical intensive care unit<br>    3. Post coronary artery bypass graft patients<br>    4. Other patients in the surgical intensive care unit<br>    5. Acute stroke patients<br>    6. General medicine ward patients<br>    7. General surgical ward patients<br>  B.  Include any of the following interventions:<br>    1. Continuous IV insulin infusion<br>    2. GIK, GI<br>    3. SQ insulin:  sliding scale v. basal bolus<br>  C.  Examine any of the following endpoints:<br>    1. Final outcomes:  mortality; cardiovascular events; CHF; disability (neuro-disability score); wound infection; sepsis; renal failure requiring HD<br>    2. Intermediate outcomes:  glucose level; length of stay; renal failure not requiring HD<br>    3. Adverse effects – rates of hypoglycemia (any study design)<br>  D.  To address KQ3, applied rigorous methodology (controlled clinical trials including RCTs) |
| I | Include | Unpublished research meeting I1 criteria |
| I | Include | Other (specify) |
| X1 | Exclude | Study outcome does not meet I1 criteria – effects on nursing staff of IV-insulin infusion protocols, e.g. |
| X2 | Exclude | Study population does not meet criteria |
| X3 | Exclude | Type of intervention not within scope of review |
| X4 | Exclude | Other (specify) |
| X5 | Exclude | Non-English language, no abstract |
| X6 | Exclude | Non-human, animal |
| X7 | Exclude | Study design or publication type not applicable; no data |
| X8 | Exclude | Non-systematic review or background article; poor-quality systematic review |
| X9 | Exclude | Publication year outside of review time frame |
| X10 | Exclude | Duplicate publication, subgroup analysis, or extension of already included parent study – these papers will be re-examined and abstracted along with parent study |

# APPENDIX C.    USPSTF QUALITY RATING CRITERIA

## Randomized Controlled Trials (RCTs) and Cohort Studies
### Criteria

- Initial assembly of comparable groups:  RCTs—adequate randomization, including concealment and whether potential confounders were distributed equally among groups; cohort studies—consideration of potential confounders with either restriction or measurement for adjustment in the analysis; consideration of inception cohorts

- Maintenance of comparable groups (includes attrition, cross-overs, adherence, contamination)

- Important differential loss to follow-up or overall high loss to follow-up

- Measurements: equal, reliable, and valid (includes masking of outcome assessment)

- Clear definition of interventions

- Important outcomes considered

- Analysis: adjustment for potential confounders for cohort studies, or intention-to-treat analysis for RCTs (i.e. analysis in which all participants in a trial are analyzed according to the intervention to which they were allocated, regardless of whether or not they completed the intervention)

### Definition of ratings based on above criteria

Good:    Meets all criteria: Comparable groups are assembled initially and maintained throughout the study (follow-up at least 80 percent); reliable and valid measurement instruments are used and applied equally to the groups; interventions are spelled out clearly; important outcomes are considered; and appropriate attention to confounders in analysis.

Fair:    Studies will be graded "fair" if any or all of the following problems occur, without the important limitations noted in the "poor" category below: Generally comparable groups are assembled initially but some question remains whether some (although not major) differences occurred in follow-up; measurement instruments are acceptable (although not the best) and generally applied equally; some but not all important outcomes are considered; and some but not all potential confounders are accounted for.

Poor:    Studies will be graded "poor" if any of the following major limitations exists: Groups assembled initially are not close to being comparable or maintained throughout the study; unreliable or invalid measurement instruments are used or not applied at all equally among groups (including not masking outcome assessment); and key confounders are given little or no attention.

# APPENDIX D    REVIEWER COMMENTS AND RESPONSES

| Reviewer | Comment | Response |
|---|---|---|
| **GENERAL COMMENTS** | | |
| **Question 1. Is the report well structured and organized?** | | |
| Aron | (Strongly agree, no comment) | Noted |
| Pogach | (Strongly agree) Follows agreed upon format | Noted |
| Ahmann | agree | Noted |
| **Question 2. Are the main points clearly presented?** | | |
| Aron | (Strongly agree, no comment) | Noted |
| Pogach | (Strongly agree) Review of methodological shortcomings of available studies, and paucity of data appropriate | Noted |
| Ahmann | agree | Noted |
| **Question 3. Is the report relevant to clinical practice?** | | |
| Aron | (Strongly agree, no comment) | Noted |
| Pogach | (Strongly agree) Yes. This report is quite relevant to clinical practice. Hope that it gets published. | Noted |
| Ahmann | disagree | Noted |
| **Question 4. Did the summary reflect the main points of the report?** | | |
| Aron | (Strongly agree, no comment) | Noted |
| Pogach | (Strongly agree, no comment) | Noted |
| Ahmann | (Agree) | Noted |
| **SCOPE AND TOPIC DEVELOPMENT** | | |
| **Question 1. Are the target patient populations explicitly defined?** | | |
| Aron | (Strongly agree, no comment) | Noted |
| Pogach | (Strongly agree, no comment) | Noted |
| Ahmann | (Agree) | Noted |
| **Question 2. Is the scope of the report clearly defined?** | | |
| Aron | (Strongly agree, no comment) | Noted |
| Pogach | (Strongly agree, no comment) | Noted |
| Ahmann | (Agree) | Noted |
| **Question 3. Are the key questions important and relevant?** | | |
| Aron | (Strongly agree, no comment) | Noted |
| Pogach | (Strongly agree, no comment) | Noted |
| Ahmann | (Disagree) | Noted |
| **Question 4. Are important clinical interventions or outcomes missing?** | | |
| Aron | no | Noted |
| Pogach | (No response) | Noted |
| Ahmann | This is a very difficult topic area to review and make conclusions that are relevant. I think there was inadequate attention given to the type of protocol used, the abillity to reachgoal, and the adherence to the protocol. This last point is seldom mentioned but is clearly a problem. | Tables 1, 2, and 3 detail both the glucose targets as well as glucose levels achieved. We've added footnotes to Table 4 that detail the type of protocol used, and the data used to titrate insulin in each protocol. Table 5 and key questions 2 and 3 have been expanded and explore insulin infusion protocol studies in greater detail. In key question 3 and the discussion, we underscore the variability across protocols. |

| Reviewer | Comment | Response |
|----------|---------|----------|
| | | In discussing the discrepancy in results between the Van den Berghe SICU trials and subsequent trials we acknowledge that protocol/staffing/institutional characteristics may be responsible. We disagree that this variability makes it difficult to make relevant conclusions. We discuss the view that this discrepancy in results may highlight feasibility issues with protocol implementation and may hamper broad generalizability of single-center trial results. |

**Question 5. Is the analytic framework useful in explaining the logic and organization of the evidence report?**

| Reviewer | Comment | Response |
|----------|---------|----------|
| Aron | (Strongly agree, no comment) | Noted |
| Pogach | (Agree, no comment) | Noted |
| Ahmann | (Agree) | Noted |

**METHODS**

**Question 1. Are the methods clearly stated?**

| Reviewer | Comment | Response |
|----------|---------|----------|
| Aron | (Strongly agree, no comment) | Noted |
| Pogach | (Strongly agree, no comment) | Noted |
| Ahmann | (Agree) However, it isn't clear why unpublished studies (without peer review) were included unless they supported the contention of the authors. | We only included unpublished studies if the authors provided either a full manuscript or enough information to quality rate the study. In essence, our critical analysis of these studies provides a peer review. This approach is accepted by peer reviewed journals - in fact, a meta-analysis on inpatient glycemic control in critically ill patients just published in JAMA included many of the same unpublished studies. |

**Question 2. Are the methods for identifying relevant articles adequate?**

| Reviewer | Comment | Response |
|----------|---------|----------|
| Aron | (Strongly agree, no comment) | Noted |
| Pogach | (Strongly agree, no comment) | Noted |
| Ahmann | (disagree) I believe there are other articles that are relevant to hypoglycemia where the outcomes are not the primary measure for the study. In other words, the frequency of hypoglycemia is likely related to diagnosis but is also related to the virtues of the protocol used. Many of the European research studies cited used the Van den Berghe protocol for delivering insulin. This is very likely an inferior protocol and requires a lot of nursing experience to use properly. Yet, the frequency of hypoglycemia in Braithwaites work or that of the Yale group, where the goal of the effort was to find a more effective insulin infusion protocol, was not reported and would be very pertinent. The same is true for computerized algorithms which were not addressed in the second and third questions. | We've expanded our discussion of these issues. See Table 5 and discussion in key questions 2 and 3. |

**Question 3. Are the methods for exclusion of studies appropriate?**

| Reviewer | Comment | Response |
|----------|---------|----------|
| Aron | (Disagree) I think that exclusion criteria that result in the exclusion of the Furnery paper (ref. 84) are too narrow. I do appreciate that the paper was discussed, though. | We have added a section presenting the results and discussing strengths/weaknesses of several frequently cited observational trials including the Furnary paper. |
| Pogach | (Agree) The Furnary article is not randomized, but does trend improved outcomes with improved glycemic control over time, including subsequent to the implementation of the infusion. The question for me is whether or not this study sufficiently controls for other contributing factors to infections and mortality to permit a conclusion that glycemic control is an independent factor. I would prefer to see the study included and critiqued in greater detail, although I understand the rationale for exclusion. | See above<br>We expanded our discussion of Furnary. The issue that most weakens the strength of conclusions from these studies derives from the use of historic controls. Observational studies, especially those that do not use prospective control groups, may overestimate treatment benefit. Though Furnary et al do attempt to control for severity of illness, it is possible that additional confounding factors were not accounted for. Moreover, it is very possible that regression to the mean and the effects of secular improvements in surgical and ICU care may account for a |

| Reviewer | Comment | Response |
|---|---|---|
| | | substantial proportion of the outcome improvement observed in the study. |
| Ahmann | agree | Noted |

**Question 4. Are the methods for grading the quality of individual studies appropriate?**

| Reviewer | Comment | Response |
|---|---|---|
| Aron | (Agree, no comment) | Noted |
| Humphrey | my biggest suggestion is that somehow you need to be more transparent about your quality ratings. if you have a quality table that you can include or if you can add a few qualtiy columns to your evidence tables that might be helpful. you can also just add a quality column and then use foot notes to indicate where it fell down in quality. i like a real qualtiy table much better tho. | We will include our quality table as an appendix and we will describe major reasons for downgrading of quality scores in the Results section. |
| Pogach | No response | Noted |
| Ahmann | (disagree) Studies that are not completed due to their inability to enroll to the levels indicated by power calculations should not be weighted highly, if even reported. For example, the DIGAMI II study was clearly stopped because they couldn't recruit (personal communication with the PI) and when they went to the multi-center approach to get a robust study, the investigators did a very poor job of getting to goal. Yet, the DIGAMI I and II trials were judged of equivalent quality. In fact, you gave far too much weight to trials where the study was stopped early and the power to make a conclusion was lost. Yet, you included those studies in your interpretation of the questions. | We do now make a note of studies that were stopped early for reasons other then benefit or harm. We believe the studies are still relevant to the questions. The inclusion of other trials that were stopped early because of benefit or harm (eg - the VISEP study) we believe is justifiable because the finding of excess harm is an important finding that, if the trials are similar internally valid, should be given equal weight. Furthermore, the use of meta-analysis for the ICU studies should help improve power to detect a difference if one existed. |

**RESULTS - BY KEY QUESTION**

*Key Question 1. Does strict glycemic control compared to less strict glycemic control improve final health outcomes in the following patients?*

**Question 1. Is the amount of detail presented in this screening key question appropriate?**

| Reviewer | Comment | Response |
|---|---|---|
| Aron | (Agree) | Noted |
| Pogach | Very well documented | Noted |
| Ahmann | (Agree) | Noted |

**Question 2. Are the summary and evidence tables clear, and/or do they highlight the main issues?**

| Reviewer | Comment | Response |
|---|---|---|
| Humphrey | I believe you need a little more detail in your evidence tables. | We are adding a column to in-text tables detailing concomitant nutrition/therapy. Our larger parent evidence tables are available for review upon request. |
| Aron | (Agree) | Noted |
| Ahmann | (disagree) When you agree that the GIK protocols (where glucose control was not a target) were not of benefit, how can you include them with the other protocols in deciding benefit of IIP in CABG patients. Furthermore, the Gandhi article is a study of the impact of the couple hours intra-operatively and should not be considered as an overall study of glucose control peri-operatively. These patients were all treated very aggressively after they left the OR. Also, you included far too many studies that were small (<400 patients and frequently < 100 patients) that in this format neutralize the effect of much larger studies.<br><br>Your discussion on page 19 is very biased and concerns me about the slant on the rest of the work. How can you report the results separately without the Van den Berghe results as "most directly addressing the question of efficacy" when other studies included in that meta-analysis had flaws that were greater. | We included GIK studies if they used a glucose target. We attempted to clarify this - in the last paragraph of the perioperative section, we list all the references we excluded because the intervention did not use a glucose target. We agree that the Gandhi study examines a different time-frame for glucose control, but we do clearly note this in the text and table and we do not believe the inclusion of this study diminishes the conclusion that the body of literature examining perioperative glucose control is heterogenous, methodologically limited, and does not provide clear evidence of benefit from tight glycemic control in perioperative settings.<br>In terms of the size of the studies - there were no larger studies that met inclusion criteria for the perioperative subsection and this again supports the conclusion that there is limited evidence in perioperative settings.<br>Re: the discussion of meta-analysis results excluded Van den Berghe - we attempted to clarify the language used in the text. Essentially, excluding Van den Berghe from the meta-analysis |

| Reviewer | Comment | Response |
|---|---|---|
| **Question 3. What evidence have we included that ought to be excluded or down-weighted?** | | |
| Pogach | None. | Noted |
| Ahmann | The VISEP study was one of the few studies you rated as "good quality" but it ended far short of its power calculation (<<50%) and was actually performed using the Van den berghe protocol. I don't understand why this study was considered better evidence than Van den Berghe's studies. You can make conclusions about hypoglycemia for this and the GLUCONTROL but you must consider the quality of their IIP and its implementation. You cannot comment on results when these studies were not powered to find such differences in the number of patients they had at completion. | We agree about the quality rating issues and we've re-evaluated all studies. We agree that the power issues for studies stopped early need to be discussed, but we disagree that results from these studies cannot be included. To help address some of these concerns we;ve added a meta-analysis of ICU studies. We discuss the power issue in the methods section as a rationale for performing meta-analysis of the ICU studies and in the discussion section as well. In terms of stopping rules and consequent power issues: the Van den Berghe SICU trial was actually also stopped short of its original recruitment goals and there is some literature suggesting that studies stopped early for benefit may overestimate treatment effects - we've added this to our discussion as well. |
| **Question 4. Do you know of studies we have overlooked?** | | |
| Aron | no | Noted |
| Pogach | No. | Noted |

*Key Question 2. What are the harms of strict glycemic control in the above subpopulations?*

| Reviewer | Comment | Response |
|---|---|---|
| **Question 1. Is the amount of detail presented in this treatment key question appropriate?** | | |
| Aron | (Agree) | Noted |
| Pogach | (Strongly agree) | Noted |
| Ahmann | (Agree) | Noted |
| **Question 2. Are the summary and evidence tables clear, and/or do they highlight the main issues?** | | |
| Aron | (Agree) | Noted |
| Pogach | (Strongly agree) | Noted |
| Ahmann | (disagree) More attention to the type of infusion protocol should be included to identify infusion protocols with greater risk. Also, why are some studies included on the tables referring to "frequency of hypoglycemia" when they don't include rates of hypoglycemia? In the hypoglycemia table on "observational studies" the Krinsley experience is listed twice when one patient population is probably a subset of the other. Why are not the Goldberg articles (Yale) and North Carolina (Braithwaite) and several studies from Atlanta not included in the observational group? They are good protocols (probably far superior to the Van den Berghe protocol used in GLUCONTROL, VISEP and others). | Please see comments above under scope and topic development. Originally we had intended to use existing systematic reviews as the basis for key question 3. Given the appropriate concern that more emphasis should be placed on the protocols themselves, we've added a number of studies to Table 5 (including the Goldberg and Braithwaite studies). |
| **Question 3. What evidence have we included that ought to be excluded or down-weighted?** | | |
| Pogach | None. | Noted |
| **Question 4. Do you know of studies we have overlooked?** | | |
| Aron | no | Noted |
| Pogach | no | Noted |

*Key Question 3. What are the most effective and safest means of lowering blood glucose in the above subpopulations?*

| Reviewer | Comment | Response |
|---|---|---|
| **Question 1. Is the amount of detail presented in this key question appropriate?** | | |
| Aron | (Disagree) details about similarities and differences among the protocols would be useful. | We will add more detail to the Key Question 3 section when describing the two systematic reviews upon which this discussion is based. |
| Pogach | (Strongly agree) | Noted |
| Ahmann | (agree) | Noted |
| **Question 2. What evidence have we included that ought to be excluded or down-weighted?** | | |
| Pogach | None | Noted |

| Reviewer | Comment | Response |
|---|---|---|
| Humphrey | You probably need to be more clear how you came up with only 5 observational studies in the harms section. those studies look highly suspicious to me for selection bias. their rates of hypoglycemia are not believeable. i recommend leaving out the observational studies since you ahve a lot of trial data. regarding the hypoglycemia, you may want to add more to the text about the degree of hypoglycemia most studies counted. it seems fairly extreme. my guess is that there was a lot of hypoglycemia in the 60 80 range. | We had excluded several observational studies because they reported hypoglycemia rates per number of glucose measurements rather than per person. We will clarify this in the text, reference these additional studies and also present their rates of hypoglycemia (while making it clear that reported rates use different denominators). We do think that it is appropriate to include observational trials for the harms question as these trials add information about "real-life" utility of these protocols. In terms of the definition of hypoglycemia in each study, this information is presented in a column within the in-text hypoglycemia table. |
| Ahmann | No discussion of computerized models or the different types of protocols that have been used. | Two studies met inclusion and are added to Table 5 and we also mention this as an area for future research. |

## Question 3. Do you know of studies we have overlooked?

| | | |
|---|---|---|
| Pogach | None | Noted |

## CONCLUSIONS AND FUTURE RESEARCH

## Question 1. Are the implications of the major findings clearly stated?

| | | |
|---|---|---|
| Aron | strongly agree | Noted |
| Pogach | strongly agree | Noted |
| Ahmann | (disagree) I think there should be more emphasis on the real questions that are raised by the studies that have been done. One would come out concluding that the evidence says intensive insulin therapy in the hospital is not supported by the literature but the literature is inadequate.<br>I think the real questions are<br>What should the target be?<br>What types of approaches help us to get there safely and effectively?<br>Importantly, the recent studies that failed to show a benefit of intensive control compared the "intensive group" to a level of control that is actually quite good. The glucose level sought in the control group is much better than the standard of the past. Furthermore, these were not completed studies. Maybe the goal should be 100–150 but that is not determined by any of the studies.<br>Also, how long does it take to get to goal? How much glucose variability is there when you get to goal? How much of this is due to nursing error because of poor inservice education or complexity of the protocol? These and many other questions are important? Obviously it is not black and white when you consider all of the permutations of the studies that have been done. | We agree that the literature to date does not answer what the glucose target should be. We suggest that the literature to date does not support widespread application of a normal glucose target in ICU patients as has been supported in some guideline recommendations. We tried to clarify in our discussion and conclusion that the literature simply does not tell us much about higher targets. The conclusion reads as follows: The use of intensive insulin therapy to achieve normoglycemia in critically ill patients does not clearly result in health outcome benefits and is associated with high rates of hypoglycemia. More moderate blood glucose control to targets above the normoglycemic range can likely be safely achieved, though the health outcome benefit of this practice has not been well studied.<br>Re: variability issues - discussed in several comments above. We added some language to key question 3 and the discussion suggesting that this variabilitiy underscores the complexity of instituting insulin infusion protocols. |

## Question 2. Has the evidence report dealt adequately with the gaps in the literature?

| | | |
|---|---|---|
| Aron | agree | Noted |
| Pogach | strongly agree | Noted |
| Ahmann | agree | Noted |

## Question 3. Does the evidence report highlight all the appropriate main conclusions and considerations for future research?

| | | |
|---|---|---|
| Aron | agree | Noted |
| Pogach | strongly agree | Noted |

## Question 4. Does the summary and benefits of harms section adequately address the issues?

| | | |
|---|---|---|
| Pogach | strongly agree | Noted |

## ADDITIONAL COMMENTS

| Reviewer | Comment | Response |
|---|---|---|
| Pogach | Page iv, line 16 section and related sections. The framing of the results is important. I would concur with the issues regarding the efficacy of "tight" control. However, the question is whether or not there is sufficient evidence to make a statement regarding improved control? As opposed to not treating hyperglycemia. | The summary paragraph at the beginning of the Key Question 1 exec summary section (page iv, lines 10–12) does say that the impact of lowering glucose to higher targets is uncertain. We will also clarify in the following paragraph that most ICU studies targeted normoglycemia. |
| Humphrey | 3. in general i think you would do well by adding a few subtitles to keep readers very clear about what you are talking about as it is easy to get lost in the detail., <br> 4. i like figure 2 alot, <br> 6. be sure to add the stroke data to table 3, ref 15.(evidence table 2?). <br> 7. you probably could add a few more outcomes to the table also if you wanted. you discuss more of them in the text than are in the table. maybe under another column. | 3 - we will add more subheadings <br> 4 - thank you <br> 6 - will add <br> 7 - some additional outcomes are mentioned under a comments heading. The parent evidence table includes all of this information. The presented tables are meant to be in-text tables, so space will be limited. |
| Render | Executive Summary, MICU/SICU: Concerns with the Brunkhorst study. 1) underpowered 2) unclear if there was a significant difference in glycemic control between the 2 groups since they only provide information about AM glucose. What about glucose values the rest of the day? Regarding the Van den Berghe studies, the bulk of mortality reduction in the SICU study came from those long-stay patients and the absolute reduction in mortality for MICU and SICU long stay patients is basically equal. | The individual studies are discussed in more detail in the full report (there simply wasn't space in the executive summary to provide all relevant information). For Brunkhorst, we clarify the number of patients included vs number projected in the results section. <br> The reporting of mean AM blood glucose was common to most of the ICU studies, including the two Van der Berghe studies. The relative decrease in AM blood glucose in Brunkhorst was comparable to the Van der Berghe SICU study. <br> The issue of the long-stay subgroup benefit is discussed in our full report. |
| Render | The trials that did indeed focus on glycemic control using adjustable dose insulin are limited by methodologic problems. One example is DIGAMI 2 which was not able, again, to establish real glycemic differences between groups, was underpowered, and randomized < 50% of patients. | We agree that there are methodologic issues that limit the strength of the conclusions and we do acknowledge this in the exec summary ("...but variation in trial design, achievement of recruitment goals, glucose level achieved, and concomitant therapy for MI limit the strength of this conclusion."). These limitations are further detailed in the full report. |
| Render | Executive Summary, CABG: The Gandhi study was looking at intraoperative control. ALL patients received glycemic control post-operatively. So the intervention lasted a few hours. The study was not powered to show a difference in mortality and it would be expected that a few hours of glycemic control beyond the tight control that all patients already receive post-op would not make a difference. | We agree that the Gandhi study (and others) were likely underpowered to show differences in final health outcomes and this is acknowledged in the exec summary and full report. The study details are presented in the full report. We will clarify in the report that this study was really designed to look at the effect of intraoperative control on patient outcomes. We do believe the outcomes as reported are still important to present while acknowledging the contextual methodologic considerations. |
| Render | Key Question 3: I have attached a reference list (some studies, some just opinion or review) addressing sliding scale. The Queale and Umpierrez studies suggest sliding scale monotherapy is not safe or effective. | Thank you for the reference list. We relied on two recent systematic reviews for our key question 3 discussion. We agree that limited evidence suggests basal-bolus regimens may be more effective than sliding scale. We do present more detail in the body of the report and will add additional references if there are controlled clinical trials examining sliding scale insulin that we missed. |
| Render | The overall limitation of this position statement/summary is that in answering question #1, it ignores data from well conducted observational studies suggesting that hyperglycemia is harmful (especially for AMI). The problem with relying on RCTs that attempt to address whether glycemic control in the ICU is beneficial is that most trials, even multi-center studies, have been ineffective due to difficulty achieving adequate power and/or establishing glycemic differences between study groups. | In our introduction, we do report there is a body of evidence suggesting an association between hyperglycemia and poor outcomes in various inpatient subpopulations. We disagree that this body of evidence (eg - the Capes systematic reviews) can be extrapolated to answer the question of whether or not intervening with intensive insulin therapy will result in improved outcomes. In terms of evaluating other observational trials that examine the effects of intensive insulin therapy, there are several that are frequently cited and will be discussed in the revised report. |

| Reviewer | Comment | Response |
|---|---|---|
| Barrett | 1. Some of the questions, e.g. Key Q 1 subpopulation any ward patient, and Key Q 3 did not require a systematic review to answer as there is almost no data. Consideration in highlighting this including not having them as questions may be given. I would be concerned about mis-interpretation of results and importance with repeated mentioning of these categories throughout the document giving them as much weight it would seem at times as the other Key Qs that did have data. | We agree there are limited data in these subpopulations. The key questions were developed based on input from those commissioning the report. In situations in which there are limited data, we believe that clearly defining the limitations of the literature after a systematic search may help direct future research efforts and clinical applicability of currently available data. |
| Barrett | 2. The different inclusion criteria for Key Q 2 (Harm) makes the document biased by definition. Data is just data, why not treat all the questions the same? The issue of harm in particular is controversial, so I understand why you would want to include more obs data, but then why not include the same quality obs data for the rest of the Qs? | There are numerous precedents for using observational data to investigate harms in systematic reviews and our current methods manual supports this approach when efficacy studies don't adequately address harms. In this case, we felt investigating hypoglycemia rates in observational studies (and trials without health outcomes) would also contribute valuable information about the feasibility of IIT in various settings since hypoglycemia is |
| Barrett | 3. The reference to Furary I believe is this: Zerr KJ, Furnary AP, Grunkemeier GL, Bookin S, Kanhere V, Starr A. Glucose control lowers the risk of wound infection in diabetics after open heart operations. Ann Thorac Surg. 1997 Feb;63(2):356–6. Your reference was from 2006. As we discussed, this paper in 1997 (over 10 years ago) started the entire inpatient tight glycemic control movement. The systematic review should dwell more on this paper and perhaps state that if you were to include the data from this paper it would/would not change your recommendation. It is a cultural thing and will be a major critique of the systematic review unless you address it fully. | See above - we expanded our discussion of Furnary and other observational studies. The references chosen contributed the most up-to-date data from the studies. |
| Ahmann | I realize this is a very difficult process and the studies are really not comparable. They have different populations, use different tools that vary in complexity and effectiveness, report different outcomes (including variable ways of reporting glucose and hypoglycemia rates), and probably represent highly variable nursing performance for utilizing the protocols properly.<br><br>I personally don't think the goal is 110 mg/dl but we have to be careful not to leave the impression that inattention to glucose control is the goal supported by the evidence. Highlighting the limitations of studies and trying to find those few things that we can conclude should be the most clear messages. For example, GIK infusions are not useful. The studies don't help us determine the optimal goals. Period! | The report was commissioned to determine the state of the evidence and is not intended to serve as a clinical guideline. We agree that ultimately, implementation decisions will need to take into account the variability in practice (eg - acknowledge local nursing performance/resources etc). |

## Reviewers

| | |
|---|---|
| Ahmann | Andrew Ahmann, MD |
| Aron | David Aron, MD |
| Barrett | Tom Barrett, MD |
| Humphrey | Linda Humphrey, MD, MPH |
| Pogach | Leonard Pogach, MD |
| Render | Marta Render, MD |

# APPENDIX E   TABLE OF QUALITY RATINGS

| Author, Year (ref) | Random assignment? | Allocation concealed? | Groups similar at baseline? | Eligibility criteria specified? | Blinding: outcome assessors, care provider, patient? | Intention-to-treat analysis? | Maintenance of comparable groups? | Reporting of attrition, contamination etc? |
|---|---|---|---|---|---|---|---|---|
| Arabi1 | yes | yes | yes | yes | NR (outcomes assessors) no (care providers) | yes | yes | yes |
| Azevedo, 20072 | yes | NR | yes | yes | NR | yes | yes | NR |
| Bilotta, 20073 | yes | yes | yes | yes | no | yes | NR | yes |
| Brunkhorst, 20084 | yes | yes | Yes | Yes | NR (outcomes assessors) no (care providers) | yes | yes | yes |
| Butterworth, 20055 | Yes | NR | Yes | Yes | Subjects yes; study nurse not blinded (adjusted insulin rates) | Yes | Yes | Yes |
| Ceremuzyski, 19996 | yes | yes | yes | yes | NR | yes | yes | yes |
| Cheung, 20067 | yes | yes | yes | yes | NR no (care providers) | yes | yes | yes |
| Diaz, 20078 | yes | yes | yes | yes | no (care providers) | yes | yes | yes |

| Author, Year (ref) | Random assignment? | Allocation concealed? | Groups similar at baseline? | Eligibility criteria specified? | Blinding: outcome assessors, care provider, patient? | Intention-to-treat analysis? | Maintenance of comparable groups? | Reporting of attrition, contamination etc? |
|---|---|---|---|---|---|---|---|---|
| Farah, 2007[9] | yes | NR | No: intervention group with lower day 1 glucose, and trend towards more DM2 in control group although did not reach stat sig. | Yes, excluded patients with stay < 3 days, but does not report how many | NR | NR | NR | NR |
| Gandhi, 2007[10] | yes | yes | Yes | Yes | Patients no; care providers no; outcome assessors yes. | No; 7-8 pts in each group were excluded because BG <100 mg/dL | Yes | Yes |
| Gray, 2007[11] | yes | yes | yes | yes | yes (outcomes assessors) no (care providers) | yes | yes | yes Moderate attrition - approx 80% were in per-protocol dataset at 90 days (I = 76.3, C = 85.3) |
| Grey, 2004[12] | Yes | NR | Yes | Yes, but not well defined and number included compared to number eligible not reported | NR | NR | NR | NR |
| Krljanac, 2005[13] | yes | yes | yes | yes | no | yes | yes | yes |
| Lazar, 2004[14] | Yes | NR | Yes | Yes | No | Yes | Yes | Yes, none |
| Li, 2006[15] | Yes but method not described | Unclear | Yes | Yes | Not blinded | No. 7 who switched Tx were excluded from analysis | Unclear | Yes. 7 switched from SQI to CII |
| Mackenzie[16] | yes | yes | No - significantly higher proportion of liver | yes, but did not specify how anticipated LOS > 48 | no | yes | yes | yes |

| Author, Year (ref) | Random assignment? | Allocation concealed? | Groups similar at baseline? | Eligibility criteria specified? | Blinding: outcome assessors, care provider, patient? | Intention-to-treat analysis? | Maintenance of comparable groups? | Reporting of attrition, contamination etc? |
|---|---|---|---|---|---|---|---|---|
| | | | disease in control group | hours was defined | | | | |
| Malmberg, 199517 | yes | yes | yes | yes | NR no (care providers) | yes | yes | yes |
| Malmberg, 200518 | yes | NR | no - control group had fewer patients with h/o prior MI | yes | NR | yes | yes | NR |
| Mehta, 200519 | yes | yes | yes | yes | yes (outcomes assessors) NR (care providers) | yes | yes | yes |
| Oksanen, 200720 | yes | yes | yes | yes | NR (assessors) no (care providers) | yes | yes | yes |
| Pache, 200421 | yes | NR | yes | yes | NR | yes | NR | NR |
| Preiser22 | yes | yes | yes | yes | yes (outcome assessors) no (care providers) | yes | yes | yes |
| Rasoul, 200723 | yes | NR | yes | yes | no | yes | yes | yes |
| Smith, 200224 | yes | NR | yes | yes | NR | yes | yes | yes |

| Author, Year (ref) | Random assignment? | Allocation concealed? | Groups similar at baseline? | Eligibility criteria specified? | Blinding: outcome assessors, care provider, patient? | Intention-to-treat analysis? | Maintenance of comparable groups? | Reporting of attrition, contamination etc? |
|---|---|---|---|---|---|---|---|---|
| Turel, 200525 | reported as randomized, but appears as though assignment to groups was consecutive | no | yes | not clearly | NR | NR | yes | NR |
| van den Berghe, 200126 | yes | yes | yes | yes | yes (outcome assessors) no (care providers) | yes | yes | yes |
| Van den Berghe, 200627 | yes | Yes | yes | Yes | yes - only for clinical cause of ICU death no (care providers) | yes | yes | yes |
| van der Horst, 200328 | yes | NR | yes | yes | NR | yes | yes | NR |

## References in Quality Ratings Table

1. Arabi YM, Dabbagh OC, Tamim HM, et al. Intensive versus conventional Insulin therapy: a randomized controlled trial in medical and surgical critically ill patients. Accepted for publication. [PubMed: 18936702]
2. Azevedo JRAd, Lima ERM, Cossetti RJD, Azevedo RPd. Intensive insulin therapy versus conventional glycemic control in patients with acute neurological injury: a prospective controlled trial. Arquivos de Neuro-Psiquiatria. 2007 Sep;65(3B):733–738. [PubMed: 17952272]
3. Bilotta F, Spinelli A, Giovannini F, Doronzio A, Delfini R, Rosa G. The effect of intensive insulin therapy on infection rate, vasospasm, neurologic outcome, and mortality in neurointensive care unit after intracranial aneurysm clipping in patients with acute subarachnoid hemorrhage: a randomized prospective pilot trial. Journal of Neurosurgical Anesthesiology. 2007 Jul;19(3):156–160. [PubMed: 17592345]
4. Brunkhorst FM, Engel C, Bloos F, et al. Intensive Insulin Therapy and Pentastarch Resuscitation in Severe Sepsis. New England Journal of Medicine. 2008 January 10, 2008;358(2):125–139. [PubMed: 18184958]
5. Butterworth J, Wagenknecht LE, Legault C, et al. Attempted control of hyperglycemia during cardiopulmonary bypass fails to improve neurologic or neurobehavioral outcomes in patients without diabetes mellitus undergoing coronary artery bypass grafting. Journal of Thoracic & Cardiovascular Surgery. 2005 Nov;130(5):1319. [PubMed: 16256784]
6. Ceremuzyski L, Budaj A, Czepiel A, et al. Low-dose glucose-insulin-potassium is ineffective in acute myocardial infarction: results of a randomized multicenter Pol-GIK trial. Cardiovascular Drugs & Therapy. 1999 May;13(3):191–200. [PubMed: 10439881]
7. Cheung NW, Wong VW, McLean M. The Hyperglycemia: Intensive Insulin Infusion in Infarction (HI-5) study: a randomized controlled trial of insulin infusion therapy for myocardial infarction. Diabetes Care. 2006 Apr;29(4):765–770. [PubMed: 16567812]
8. Diaz R, Goyal A, Mehta SR, et al. Glucose-insulin-potassium therapy in patients with ST-segment elevation myocardial

infarction. JAMA. 2007 Nov 28;298(20):2399–2405. [PubMed: 18042917]

9.  Farah R, Samokhvalov A, Zviebel F, Makhoul N. Insulin therapy of hyperglycemia in intensive care. Israel Medical Association Journal: Imaj. 2007 Mar;9(3):140–142. [PubMed: 17402320]

10. Gandhi GY, Nuttall GA, Abel MD, et al. Intensive intraoperative insulin therapy versus conventional glucose management during cardiac surgery: a randomized trial. Annals of Internal Medicine. 2007 Feb 20;146(4):233–243. [PubMed: 17310047]

11. Gray CS, Hildreth AJ, Sandercock PA, et al. Glucose-potassium-insulin infusions in the management of post-stroke hyperglycaemia: the UK Glucose Insulin in Stroke Trial (GIST-UK). Lancet Neurology. 2007 May;6(5):397–406. [PubMed: 17434094]

12. Grey NJ, Perdrizet GA. Reduction of nosocomial infections in the surgical intensive-care unit by strict glycemic control. Endocrine Practice. 2004 Mar-Apr;10( Suppl 2):46–52. [PubMed: 15251640]

13. Krljanac G, Vasiljevi Z, Radovanovi M, et al. Effects of glucose-insulin-potassium infusion on ST-elevation myocardial infarction in patients treated with thrombolytic therapy. American Journal of Cardiology. 2005 Oct 15;96(8):1053–1058. [PubMed: 16214437]

14. Lazar HL, Chipkin SR, Fitzgerald CA, Bao Y, Cabral H, Apstein CS. Tight glycemic control in diabetic coronary artery bypass graft patients improves perioperative outcomes and decreases recurrent ischemic events. Circulation. 2004 Mar 30;109(12):1497–1502. [PubMed: 15006999]

15. Li J-Y, Sun S, Wu S-J. Continuous insulin infusion improves postoperative glucose control in patients with diabetes mellitus undergoing coronary artery bypass surgery. Texas Heart Institute Journal. 2006;33(4):445–451. [PMC free article: PMC1764949] [PubMed: 17215967]

16. Mackenzie IM, Blunt M, Ingle S, Palmer CR. GLYcaemic Control and Outcome in GENeral Intensive Care: The East Anglian GLYCOGENIC study. Unpublished report.

17. Malmberg K, Ryden L, Efendic S, et al. Randomized trial of insulin-glucose infusion followed by subcutaneous insulin treatment in diabetic patients with acute myocardial infarction (DIGAMI study): effects on mortality at 1 year. Journal of the American College of Cardiology. 1995 Jul;26(1):57–65. [PubMed: 7797776]

18. Malmberg K, Ryden L, Wedel H, et al. Intense metabolic control by means of insulin in patients with diabetes mellitus and acute myocardial infarction (DIGAMI 2): effects on mortality and morbidity. European Heart Journal. 2005 Apr;26(7):650–661. [PubMed: 15728645]

19. Mehta SR, Yusuf S, Diaz R, et al. Effect of glucose-insulin-potassium infusion on mortality in patients with acute ST-segment elevation myocardial infarction: the CREATE-ECLA randomized controlled trial. JAMA. 2005 Jan 26;293(4):437–446. [PubMed: 15671428]

20. Oksanen T, Skrifvars MB, Varpula T, et al. Strict versus moderate glucose control after resuscitation from ventricular fibrillation. Intensive Care Medicine. 2007 Dec;33(12):2093–2100. [PubMed: 17928994]

21. Pache J, Kastrati A, Mehilli J, et al. A randomized evaluation of the effects of glucose-insulin-potassium infusion on myocardial salvage in patients with acute myocardial infarction treated with reperfusion therapy. American Heart Journal. 2004 Jul;148(1):e3. [PubMed: 15215812]

22. Preiser JC.Glucontrol Study: Comparing the Effects of Two Glucose Control Regimens by Insulin in Intensive Care Unit Patients. NIH; http://www.clinicaltrials.gov/ct/gui/show/NCT00107601. Submitted for publication.

23. Rasoul S, Ottervanger JP, Timmer JR, et al. One year outcomes after glucose-insulin-potassium in ST elevation myocardial infarction. The Glucose-insulin-potassium study II. International Journal of Cardiology. 2007 Oct 31;122(1):52–55. [PubMed: 17223212]

24. Smith A, Grattan A, Harper M, Royston D, Riedel BJCJ. Coronary revascularization: a procedure in transition from on-pump to off-pump? The role of glucose-insulin-potassium revisited in a randomized, placebo-controlled study. Journal of Cardiothoracic & Vascular Anesthesia. 2002 Aug;16(4):413–420. [PubMed: 12154417]

25. Turel B, Gemici K, Baran I, et al. Effects of glucose-insulin-potassium solution added to reperfusion treatment in acute myocardial infarction. Anadolu Kardiyoloji Dergisi. 2005 Jun;5(2):90–94. [PubMed: 15939681]

26. van den Berghe G, Wouters P, Weekers F, et al. Intensive insulin therapy in the critically ill patients. New England Journal of Medicine. 2001 Nov 8;345(19):1359–1367. [PubMed: 11794168]

27. Van den Berghe G, Wilmer A, Hermans G, et al. Intensive insulin therapy in the medical ICU. New England Journal of Medicine. 2006 Feb 2;354(5):449–461. [PubMed: 16452557]

28. van der Horst ICC, Zijlstra F, van't Hof AWJ, et al. Glucose-insulin-potassium infusion inpatients treated with primary angioplasty for acute myocardial infarction: the glucose-insulin-potassium study: a randomized trial. Journal of the American College of Cardiology. 2003 Sep 3;42(5):784–791. [PubMed: 12957421]